the DR. BAZZI METHOD of IMPLANT DENTISTRY

saving

SMILES

changing

LIVES

DR. NADER BAZZI

the DR. BAZZI METHOD of IMPLANT DENTISTRY

saving

SMILES

changing

LIVES

WHERE SMILES DO COME TRUE!

Advantage®

Published by Advantage, Charleston, South Carolina.
Member of Advantage Media Group.

ADVANTAGE is a registered trademark and the Advantage colophon is a trademark of Advantage Media Group, Inc.

Printed in the United States of America.

ISBN: 978-1-59932-155-4
LCCN: 2012956250

This publication is designed to provide accurate and authoritative information in regard to the subject matter covered. It is sold with the understanding that the publisher is not engaged in rendering legal, accounting, or other professional services. If legal advice or other expert assistance is required, the services of a competent professional person should be sought.

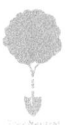
Advantage Media Group is proud to be a part of the Tree Neutral® program. Tree Neutral offsets the number of trees consumed in the production and printing of this book by taking proactive steps such as planting trees in direct proportion to the number of trees used to print books. To learn more about Tree Neutral, please visit www.treeneutral.com. To learn more about Advantage's commitment to being a responsible steward of the environment, please visit www.advantagefamily.com/green

Advantage Media Group is a leading publisher of business, motivation, and self-help authors. Do you have a manuscript or book idea that you would like to have considered for publication? Please visit www.advantagefamily.com or call 1.866.775.1696

Dedication, Gratitude, Acknowledgment

To my wife Rima, and my children, Julia and Tamer, for their love and unconditional support and for the blessed life we have. Rima, I am forever thankful for your love, beauty, and grace.

To my mom who taught me love and kindness.

To my extended family whose support is very much appreciated.

To my patients: without you this book would never have been written, your trust in me allowed me to pursue my passion. I will forever be grateful.

To my team for your dedication, grace, and compassion to profoundly enhance the quality of the lives of our patients.

Table of Contents

f o r e w o r d

---

by Gary Kadi

The Mouth

Your Source of Complete Health and Quality of Life

When Dr. Nadar Bazzi asked me to write the foreword for this profound and groundbreaking book, I was completely honored.

I have had the privilege of collaborating with thousands of doctors globally over the last eighteen years and Dr. Bazzi is a very generous man, husband, father, friend, dentist, caregiver, innovator, community leader, and humanitarian.

My connection and affinity to Dr. Bazzi and his healthcare team comes from my personal mission to have the American public understand that the mouth is the gateway to total and complete health and dental teams are the unsung heroes to complete health. We are leading a movement called the Cavity in Healthcare Reform. Dr. Bazzi's Method™ of implant dentistry is the cornerstone of this movement.

One of the most important things I can say is that Dr. Bazzi is an incredible human being first and foremost and because of that, he is one of the best practitioners on planet. He can be called the king of implantology! His ability to care deeply for humanity is what makes him an outstanding dentist.

He is highly respected by many because he deeply respects others, from honoring his wife and partner, Dr. Rima Bazzi, to nurturing his ten-year-old daughter, Julia, and his seven-year-old son, Tamer, to respecting and supporting his dental team. Dr. Bazzi naturally goes beyond what the average husband, father, and dentist can provide. His mission for Complete Health Dentistry is the driving force behind this book you're about to read. Dr. Bazzi is an indisputable leader in the Complete Health Dentistry community in the metropolitan area of Detroit, in Michigan, and nationally.

His is the example of selfless generosity. Some people are takers and hoarders and others, like Dr. Nader Bazzi, are value creators who are always asking, "How can I make this community a better place, how can I help more people, and how can I educate people that the mouth is the gateway to total health and wellness?" This is what the seed of the work you are about to experience is rooted and fertilized in.

Whether through offering free dental days for patients without the means to pay for their treatment or a commitment to re-educating the public that dentistry is not just about drilling, filling, and billing, Dr. Bazzi is progressive, and he truly understands that the mouth is the portal to total health and wellness as well as looking and feeling better about yourself. A healthy, good-looking smile is a self-confidence game changer.

In Michigan and around the nation, Dr. Bazzi is mobilizing this vital educational and scientific movement on all-sized scales. His humanitarian spirit combined with his proprietary implant methodology is solely motivated by his desire to create the best quality of life and health for people, while removing the pain and suffering of getting dental work completed and maintaining it. Dr. Bazzi understands that having a fixed solution for his patients is not only in their best interest in terms of money but also in terms of the function and maintenance of their dignity and freedom from embarrassment. This allows his patients and the other healthcare professionals he inspires to have confidence in their smile and in their health.

After all, the mouth is the source for all health. We kiss, speak, nourish ourselves, breathe, talk, laugh, communicate, and of course, smile through our mouth. Up until recently, no one was stepping up to allow the truth to be told about that.

Dr. Bazzi, along with a visionary group of men and women who understand the mouth has been neglected as part of overall healthcare reform, are now making a stand for you to understand its importance in increasing longevity and reducing high healthcare costs.

Thank you, Dr. Bazzi, for taking the "dent" out of dentistry and putting one into humanity's health and well-being.

While I'm on a roll, let me congratulate you, this book's reader, for being open to learning about how you can help yourself live a better life. Coming from very humble beginnings myself, I learned the hard way that in life we don't get what we deserve; we get what we *think* we deserve. Nothing more. Nothing less. Think of reading this book as a gift to yourself; you will raise the deserve level for the only body and mind you have been given.

Dr. Bazzi's Story

As a child, I always knew I wanted to do something in the medical profession. I also used to love taking toys apart and reassembling them into new designs. Dentistry has allowed me to combine those two early passions: I am able to provide life-changing medical services to patients while using my hands to create something developed in my own mind. However, there is another reason my work in dentistry has been so very rewarding to me: I feel a smile is an outward reflection of what's inside *you*. For me to truly help my patient—to explain the need for a service or procedure, and to do so in a way that engenders trust—that patient needs to feel my convictions about his or her care are coming from the bottom of my heart. My smile conveys an honest, positive attitude and energy that helps accomplish this goal. By restoring my patients' own smiles, I help them express their true selves and accomplish their own goals. It's a job more fulfilling than I can possibly describe.

I studied dentistry at the University of Detroit, Mercy, graduating with honors in the top third of my class. During my years in dental school, I had the privilege of completing more procedures than any other student in my class. Each time I mastered one technique, I developed the confidence that motivated me to learn another. This process led me to perform additional advanced procedures. By the time I left dental school, I wanted to do even more. I knew there was more to the profession than the basics we had learned, and I wanted to develop my knowledge to the fullest. I wanted to build up my skills to the point where I could give back to the most challenging patients—those whose teeth could not be "saved" by traditional means—what they had lost. That is where implant dentistry came in.

When I began learning the skills and techniques necessary to perform implant dentistry, these methods weren't in widespread use. In fact, one of the final lectures I attended in dental school discussed implants as an up-and-coming treatment, but one that was too complex for the students to learn much about. Once again, I was extremely fortunate: I was able to intern for two years with the world's foremost implant dentist, Dr. Carl Misch, who has a practice in Beverly Hills, Michigan, and lectures all around the world.

With Dr. Misch as my mentor, I learned about implants from the best. When I set about developing my own dental practice, I didn't just focus on implant dentistry. I also focused on treating patients with challenging conditions of all types. Not surprisingly, many patients who require implants have a longstanding fear of dentists. That fear plays a large role in the steady deterioration of patients' teeth until they can't be saved by traditional means. I love to work with fearful patients the most. Once we work together, we will be together for life.

As a provider of implant dentistry, I have found that every patient is unique. Yet one story tends to repeat itself across patient histories. This is the story of an individual who had a bad experience at the hands of a dentist. Usually, this bad experience happens during childhood. This child grows into an adult who holds on to the fear of that experience. As a result, such adults avoid other dentists. They end up not seeking dental care until they have an absolute emergency. By that time, they are in dire pain.

I have always had an avid interest in helping such patients. First, I enjoy teaching them that they can be helped—and they can receive that help without judgment. Second, I enjoy building a rapport with them and getting them to trust again. Third, I enjoy educating them about the treatment they need and the rewards they will get from pursuing it. Above all, I enjoy seeing the transformations these individuals undergo when we work together to resolve years of dental problems.

I find it incredibly powerful to work with patients who have been fearful of dentists for most of their lives, but who come in after receiving implants and give me a hug. I also find it powerful when my patients, who have been self-conscious or downright ashamed of their mouths for years, come in and give me a proud smile. As I have seen firsthand, as long as I continue giving these people good experiences, they will eventually grow out of their fear. Watching the disappearance of such fear has been one of the biggest rewards of my career. As I have witnessed over and over again, if you care for fearful patients properly, they will not be fearful any longer.

To me, dentistry is about more than treating the teeth and gums—it's about considering the whole person. Of course, a dentist needs to be medically skilled, but a dentist also needs to be compassionate. I may look into the mouth of a patient who hasn't seen a dentist in ten, twenty, or even thirty years and know what treatment is needed, but I do not know what that patient has been through in life, I do not know *why* that patient hasn't been to the dentist in so long. *I cannot judge.* Nor do I want to. Instead, what I want to do is reassure people. Many patients come to me feeling as though their situation is hopeless. It is not. I want you to know that there is hope. I am here to make you better, to make your life better, and to make you healthier. In the process, I want to get you to smile again.

Many of my patients have told me I have been successful in reaching these goals. One of the reasons that I have had this success and that patients have such positive experiences with me is my use of IV sedation. With this technique, I am able to put patients into a twilight sleep—a state in which they are totally comfortable. After coming out of this twilight sleep, the patient doesn't remember anything about the procedure that has been performed. The technique is extremely safe, and my personal record with it is outstanding. I have probably done more than seven hundred of these sedations in my career, and I have never had problems with any of them. I have used sedation for implant dentistry and for regular fillings and cleanings. I'm one of the very few dentists in Southeast Michigan to provide this type of service. What's more, through this service I have been able to turn initially fearful individuals into satisfied patients and valued friends.

To date, I have done nearly one thousand implants. I have loved the transformation I have seen in each and every patient on which these implants were performed. Scientists have been conducting research on implant procedures since the early 1960s, so we've now got over fifty years of data on those procedures. What people have found from this data is that, when done correctly, implants yield successful, predictable results in 95 percent or more of cases. My own data, based on the implants I have done in my own practice, matches these findings. In addition to having been able to match that 95 percent success rate, I often beat it.

I attribute much of this success to the training I received from Dr. Misch. However, my success also comes from my continuing commitment to learn everything I can about implants and about dentistry as a whole. I take at least fifty to a hundred credit hours of dental education every year. Michigan's state requirement is only twenty credit hours per year, but I feel that given the rapid pace of advancement in the dental field today, this amount of time is not sufficient for me to stay up-to-date with everything I need to learn to benefit my patients.

My wife and I are both dentists. We are also proud parents to two children: a girl and a boy. I took care of my son's first cavity. Yes, he had a cavity! However, he was good about having it filled, and as you might imagine, I made sure he had a positive experience. As you might also imagine, my wife and I made healthy dental habits a priority for our children from an early age. We made sure that they brushed and flossed their teeth every night and every morning, and that practice has become a solid routine for them. It is is something we have instilled in them. I hope, as is typical of a parent, that my children's lives will be successful. However, I also hope that they will both grow up to have beautiful smiles, since I know those beautiful smiles will increase the likelihood of success in their lives.

Not everyone is raised with such focused attention to dental health and the development of healthy dental habits. If you've suffered poor teeth and dental pain for years, I want you to know that it is not your fault. However, I also want you to know that you are doing yourself a disservice by living this way. You are worth more than this. Everyone has different motivators for finally seeking dental treatment. Maybe you're worried about your health or ready to hit the dating scene. Perhaps you're just tired of dealing with the anxiety—tired of listening to the little voice in the back of your head that's been telling you to tend to your teeth. Whatever your reasons for considering dental treatment, I am glad they brought you here. I can't change your past, but together we can improve your future.

CHAPTER
one

The Significance of a Healthy Smile

The Significance of a Healthy Smile

The mouth in its entirety is an important and even wondrous part of our anatomy, our emotions, our life; it is the site of our very being. When an animal loses its teeth, it cannot survive unless it is domesticated; its very existence is terminated; it dies. In the human, the mouth is the means of speaking, of expressing love, happiness and joy, anger, ill temper, or sorrow. It is the primary sex contact; hence, it is of initial import to our regeneration and survival by food and propagation. It deserves the greatest care it can receive at any sacrifice.

—Dr. F. Harold Worth

Despite advancements in the field of dentistry, many people associate dentists with pain. Some have had negative experiences with dentists in the past and retained those painful memories over the years. In contrast, others buy into an age-old reputation: In the past, before local anesthetic was invented, dentistry was admittedly more barbaric. Over the last thirty years, however, the dental profession has become highly specialized. We dentists have made enormous strides in the treatment and care of the teeth and gums. We have made equally enormous strides in the area of pain management. As a result, a competent, caring dentist is able to make patients extremely comfortable during any treatment. Yet the truth is that even today, some patients maintain a strong fear of going to the dentist. Subsequently, and sadly, they seek dental care infrequently, if at all.

According to statistics, about 50 percent of the population in the United States does not see a dentist on a regular basis. In my experience, patients whose parents were vigilant about taking proper care of their children's teeth, and who took them to a dentist who had their best needs at heart, end up having healthy teeth throughout their lives. However, each person's experience is unique—and not all patients have been so fortunate. Some people grew up without proper home care or the means to seek regular dental care. Still others had a painful dental experience in childhood and so avoided dental care in adulthood. These are the individuals who do not see a dentist regularly. Over time, their mouth problems become worse and worse, and they only seek care when they suffer emergencies or are troubled by continuous toothaches. These are the individuals who can experience serious, albeit treatable, problems later in their lives. One of the most serious is the actual loss of a tooth or teeth.

The Importance of a Radiant Smile

The blunt truth is that missing teeth impair humans both physically and psychologically. Just ask yourself the following questions:

- Do you typically hide your smile?

- If you have a missing front tooth, do you put your hand over your mouth when you smile?

- Are you missing teeth on the side?

- Do you convince yourself that these missing teeth might not show?

- Do you hold your lips a certain way so no one can see your gap?

- Do you turn away from people, if only slightly, to mask the "missing" area?

- Do you restrict your smile, holding back your biggest grin even at the happiest or funniest moments?

If you answered with even a single affirmative, you are living proof of the psychological consequences of missing teeth: Missing teeth can seriously undermine self-confidence.

Over time, the psychological costs of missing teeth can become even higher. Technically, humans are the only animals that can live at all without their teeth. But how well can they live? Even if it does not show, a single missing tooth can cause damage you can't feel or see until it is too late. That's right. Just one missing tooth can cause a cascade of events that have led millions of people to lose more teeth needlessly. Few people, if any, would dream of leaving a gap in the front of their mouth that ruins their smile. However, many will live for years with a missing tooth in the back of their mouths. In doing so, they are unknowingly harming their smiles.

Let's examine why. Mother nature designed your teeth to work together. Each tooth is designed to perform a certain function. When a member of the group is lost, more work is required from the remaining teeth. They start to shift toward the hole left by the missing tooth. The teeth on either side tilt into the empty space. The tooth above grows down. Gaps open up. More teeth shift. Your smile changes for the worse. Now your bite is thrown off. This process almost always causes what's known as a *destructive bite*.

Destructive bites are so named because of the damage they do to the body: They can cause headaches, intolerable pain in the jaw joint, and gastrointestinal problems (discussed later on). They can also place uneven pressure on teeth, thereby causing them to break or wear down rapidly. Have you ever seen someone with short front teeth? Chances are about twenty to one that a destructive bite is the cause. Clearly, destructive bites—caused by missing back teeth—ruin smiles as surely as missing front teeth do.

There's a very good reason that I mention ruined smiles again and again: Scientific research has proven that attractiveness, and an attractive smile, determine how other people perceive and treat you. Good-looking people enjoy tremendous advantages in society. Other people see them as more intelligent. Others like them better, seeing them as having more desirable personalities. Others see these attractive individuals as more persuasive, and people are more likely to help those they admire. People perceive attractive individuals as smarter, more talented, kinder, and more honest. What physical feature outranked eyes, hair, and body as most attractive to others in a recent American Dental Association survey? You guessed it: the *smile*.

For many high-level executives, salespeople, realtors, small business owners, and others who deal with the public, their mouths are how they make money. The mouth is an instrument of communication, appearance, and self-confidence that allows people to get their jobs done and help others. Could you imagine an entertainer or a celebrity who has unattractive teeth? Absolutely not. Their looks are critical to their success.

Guess what? Your looks are valuable to your success too. If you need to get others to do things, or to win them over in some way (and who does not?), an investment in your smile could be the best money you will ever spend. By safeguarding your smile, you will be more able to convince others about your way of thinking, win a promotion, make more sales, and put much more money into your pocket.

Exactly how many people have a poor self-image because of missing teeth is difficult to determine. However, it's definitely a large percentage. A crooked smile, a missing front tooth, or an uneven bite can all make people more self-conscious. They can affect people's careers and personal lives. People who have missing teeth naturally feel less attractive to the opposite sex. As I hope you saw in the short, informal quiz at the beginning of this chapter, missing teeth make you less confident in any social situation. They can make you more likely to cover up your smile, be introverted, and shy away from social interactions.

In American culture, all of us want to have straight white teeth without any spaces or gaps. When meeting somebody for the first time, the first thing you pay attention to is his or her eyes, and the second thing is his or her smile. A smile is meant to be ravishing. A smile is an investment in you. It increases your confidence. It improves your appearance and your function. As I stated earlier, I believe a beautiful smile is a reflection of who you really are. Simply put, it's a wonderful thing to have.

The Health Consequences of Missing Teeth

Missing teeth can make you *look* older, since they encourage wrinkling and sagging skin. When you lose one tooth, the bone that surrounded it begins to shrink, and if the entire set of upper or lower teeth is lost, wrinkles and creases on the face become even more pronounced. This results in greater creases, and it will definitely make you look much older. However, missing teeth can actually *make* you older by accelerating a number of processes that age the body and threaten longevity. In fact, statistically speaking, people who have lost all their teeth live about ten years less than those who retain all their teeth.

To better understand how the loss of a tooth has such a hefty impact, I want to go back to mother nature for a moment. When a tooth is lost, nature fills the gap, and the teeth adjacent to that missing tooth start shifting. The tooth behind typically shifts forward, the tooth in front shifts backward, and the opposing tooth (in the jaw above or below the missing tooth's spot) will *hypererupt* and drop down or grow up into the gap. This combination of movements does not happen overnight. It usually takes months or even years. However, as these movements happen, a bite that used to be normal ends up becoming misaligned.

A misaligned bite does not function normally, so it impacts a person's chewing and eating. The mouth marks the starting point of the digestive process. If you don't have a proper bite, you're automatically at high risk of having gastrointestinal (GI) problems. Patients without proper bites will experience more heartburn, constipation, and GI discomfort, and their risk of blockages and polyps developing in the colon will increase. In addition, people with severe misalignments can become essentially handicapped in the sense that they can't eat nutritious, healthy meals; they tend to avoid fruits and vegetables due to the discomfort they experience when chewing. They then become nutritionally depleted, which increases the likelihood of gastrointestinal problems in itself.

Discomfort associated with missing teeth impacts more than the digestive tract. Misalignment creates painful problems caused by the uneven pressure placed on teeth themselves. A tooth subjected to undue pressure will start to develop *acute sensation*, which means it will twinge. If the pressure reaches the point at which it causes trauma to the tooth, the related nerve inside becomes painful and inflamed. That inflammation necessitates a root canal or sometimes even an extraction. The end result can thus be the loss of another tooth.

In addition, once a person's bite starts becoming misaligned, the bite begins to move the person's temporomandibular joint out of whack. The temporomandibular joint connects the lower jaw to the skull. Subjection of this joint to uneven forces by a misaligned bite can result in the development of a condition called TMJ (*temporomandibular joint disorder*). TMJ can cause headaches, earaches, and facial pain, all of which often become intense. Some sufferers have been known to drug themselves to death to escape this pain. Once again, all this started with the simple process of losing a single tooth.

Research also shows that poor dental health will predispose people to other general health problems that ultimately shorten their lives. Statistics prove that the longer you keep your teeth, the longer you end up living. Researchers are starting to discover the reasons behind the shortened life expectancy associated with poor dental health. Here are just some of the things researchers are saying about how periodontal disease, the culprit behind most tooth problems, can impact the entire body's health:

- When the oral bacteria that wreak havoc on teeth and gums invade the bloodstream, the resulting inflammation can increase fatty plaque buildup in the arteries. Over time, this buildup narrows the blood vessels that "feed" the heart. Evidence also suggests that bacteria can encourage the formation of blood clots. This is bad news, since anything that obstructs normal blood flow through the coronary arteries robs the heart itself of the oxygen and nutrients it needs to keep beating. If blood flow is reduced drastically, or cut off altogether, a heart attack may result. In fact, studies indicate that people with periodontal disease are nearly twice as likely to suffer from coronary artery disease, and they have higher risks of both heart attacks and strokes (which occur when clots block blood flow to the brain) than individuals without periodontal disease.

- The oral bacteria that cause periodontal disease may also cause lung concerns when they are inhaled, or *aspirated*, into the lungs. When researchers at SUNY Buffalo analyzed twenty-one published studies on periodontal disease and lung disease, they arrived at two fascinating conclusions:

  - Several studies pointed to an association between periodontal disease and chronic obstructive pulmonary disease, or COPD.

  - Therapies aimed at reducing periodontal bacteria also reduced the amount of hospital-acquired pneumonia by an average of 40 percent.

- Periodontal disease and diabetes are connected. People with diabetes are more prone to periodontal infections (and more susceptible to many types of infections, in fact), and emerging evidence suggests the opposite may also be true. In other words, periodontal disease may make it tougher for patients with diabetes to control their blood sugar levels. Similar to the pneumonia findings described above, one study's researchers found that when diabetes patients received treatment for periodontal infections, their ability to manage their diabetes also improved.

Obviously, the mouth-body connection is an active area of investigation. More research needs to be done, and will be done, to solidify the relationships described above, along with several others. For example, there appears to be a link between rheumatoid arthritis and periodontal disease, since many patients report that their joint pain eases when their periodontal problems are resolved. Moreover, preliminary data suggesting that periodontal disease may affect pregnancy outcomes is the reason that experts now advise women to be evaluated for tooth and gum problems before they become pregnant. Recently, researchers have even discovered that people with gum disease are more likely, statistically, to have Alzheimer's disease than those whose gums and teeth are healthy. More research is required to prove the link between the two.

The bottom line is this: Take care of your teeth by having a good oral health regimen at home and seeing the dentist on a regular basis. These practices are vital both to your appearance and your overall health. The sooner you take care of an oral health problem by visiting the dentist, the more likely you are to keep those teeth in the long term. And the more likely you are to enjoy a longer, happier life.

CHAPTER
two

Traditional Tooth Replacement Methods

Their Drawbacks and Limitations

Traditional Tooth Replacement Methods

Their Drawbacks and Limitations

According to historical records, primitive forms of dentistry date back as far as 7000 BC, when bead craftsmen used their drills to treat tooth-related problems. Ancient texts reveal that dental problems were on the radar of various civilizations, from Sumeria to China to Japan, where references to "tooth worms" as a cause of cavities can be found in texts from 5000 BC. (Incredibly, this idea actually persisted until the late fourteenth century AD).

Dental treatments also existed in ancient Rome, Greece, and Egypt. Homer, Aristotle, Hippocrates, and Cornelius Celsus describe topics such as tooth eruption, tooth extraction, gum disease, and dental therapy in varying levels of detail. Egyptian records contain the first official reference to an actual dentist: The tomb of a man named Hesy-re, who died in 2600 BC, is inscribed with the phrase, "Greatest of those who deal with teeth, and of physicians." Archeologists have also found dental work in the remains of ancient Romans and Egyptians, including an ancient form of tooth restoration in which wire was used to bind together prosthetic teeth. However, the folk in these societies had no organized approach to dentistry. The people who tended to others' tooth problems invariably wore several different hats. In fact, Hesy-re himself was a scribe in addition to a dentist and a physician.

The trend of tending to dental problems on the side continued into the Middle Ages. In Europe, dental care became the responsibility of monks and the barbers who assisted them. (Barbers became assistants because they went to monasteries to shave the monks' heads. Once there, the knives and razors they used also proved handy for tooth-related tasks). However, a series of papal edicts issued in the twelfth century banned monks from letting blood, lancing abscesses, or performing tooth extractions or surgeries of any kind. At that time, barbers took over tooth care entirely; if someone had a tooth that needed desperate attention, he or she went to the barber. The same guy who cut people's hair also pulled their teeth out, using the very same implements, no less.

Dentistry finally began to gain ground as its own profession during the 1700s. During that century French dentist Claude Mouton wrote about the root canal. He described using a gold filling and post in the process. Another French expert, Pierre Fauchard, penned a landmark text titled *Le Chirurgien Dentiste (The Surgeon Dentist)*. The Royal College of Surgeons in Edinburgh offered its first lecture specifically on teeth. In a nod to dental hygiene, people began using tooth powders. These early dentifrices, which people rubbed on their teeth using a cloth or rag, could be bought at local markets and fairs. In 1760 the first medically trained dentist to practice in America sailed over from Britain and set up shop in the colonies. Notably, Paul Revere advertised his dentistry services in a Boston newspaper eight years later.

Still, during this period of rapid change, charlatanism and quackery ran rampant in dental care. In addition, only the wealthy in Europe and America could afford a real dentist or have ready access to one. For most colonials, and for many Europeans, the local blacksmith provided the most accessible services.

Back then, there *were* dentures for those rich enough to get them, and those willing to wear ill-fitting, obviously fake teeth made from ivory, porcelain, or other people's teeth (harvested from battlefields and bolted to a base). There was no such thing as reliable dental restoration. There were no antibiotics, so many people died because of tooth problems. Tooth infections grew into abscesses that traveled underneath the mouth tissue and eventually reached the brain, causing a deadly abscess. Back then, there was no anesthetic either; the patient took a shot of whiskey, and the person removing the tooth would pull it out if he or she possibly could. Admittedly, it was pretty rough back then. I am glad we weren't alive during such a time.

In the nineteenth century dentistry made a huge leap forward, and people's use of several forms of anesthesia factored enormously into making that leap. Ether, chloroform, and nitrous oxide (also known as "laughing gas," and still used in dental offices today) gained wide use in medicine. Because of anesthesia, people became more willing to have their teeth worked on and pulled, which increased the demand for more wearable prosthetic teeth. The development of vulcanite, an inexpensive and durable material (at least, during that time) meant this new demand could be met. By the end of the century people were mass-producing more affordable dentures.

The early 1900s marked a sea change in dentistry, a time when individuals started to come together and form a profession with the dedicated aim of fixing people's oral problems in a superior way. Dentists became interested in doing more than just treating or removing problematic teeth. They wanted to have more to offer patients than a mouthful of dentures. Preserving natural teeth became a new priority for them, and these dentists made advancements in prevention of dental decay and tooth loss as rapidly as they made advancements in "problem-tooth" treatment and care.

Today dental care, both at home and in the dentist's office, has traveled light years in a relatively short period of time. At-home hygiene methods and products have become so advanced that if people use them correctly, they should, ideally, only need to go to the dentist for a regular professional cleaning and checkup. Dentist-performed cleanings remove plaque and bacteria that build up even after people perform vigilant brushing and flossing. While tooth decay can happen to even the best of us, people who go to regular checkups give their dentists the chance to spot cavities early, so the problems can easily be fixed.

When dentists fix cavities, we are actually cleaning the decayed area of the tooth and replacing it with a nice piece of restoration that will support the tooth again and make it whole. If nothing is done, however, the cavity will eventually get larger and larger until it gets to the nerve and causes a toothache. The whole point of modern dentistry is to keep such things from happening: to preserve the function of existing teeth while painlessly restoring faulty teeth so patients are able to get on with their lives.

However, there are some shortcomings with traditional dentistry, some ways in which treatment isn't consistent with the professional goal of preserving existing teeth. Let me give you this scenario. When a dentist fixes a cavity, usually he or she just cleans the teeth and gives the patient a filling. However, if a patient's cavity is larger, the process can end up turning into a root canal. This occurs when the nerve on the inside of the tooth is damaged, and the dentist needs to remove the nerve. The dentist ends up crowning the tooth, or putting a cap over it. After many years of functioning, that tooth will eventually break and fracture. At this point, all the dentist can do is extract the tooth.

The limitation concerns what the dentist can do to replace the tooth. Remember, if a patient has one tooth that is out of whack, that single tooth causes a domino effect, a cascade of problems. The dentist wants to restore the tooth to its proper function, which means restoring it to its original width and height. In the case of a single tooth extraction, the dentist's traditional means of accomplishing this restoration involve creating a *bridge*. In this process, the two teeth on either side of the missing tooth are ground down into short nubs. (Much of the time, there's nothing wrong with these teeth. The dentist grinds them down to use them as support for the new teeth that will be placed over them). The dentist takes an impression of the area and sends it out to the lab. From this impression, the lab technicians make three crowns: two for the teeth that have been shortened into nubs, and a "dummy" crown in the center to replace the missing tooth. That is the bridge, which the dentist then cements into place. This is considered the standard of care. It is a form of traditional dentistry done on an everyday basis.

The bridge lasts, on average, about ten years. Eventually, one of the two teeth supporting the bridge will fail. Despite the crown that covers it, it will fracture under pressure. This fracture necessitates additional treatment. Sometimes the dentist can perform another root canal, but often the failed tooth cannot be saved. At that point, the dentist has to extract that tooth. The patient started with one lost tooth. Ten years later, he or she has two lost teeth. The process keeps going from there. A dentist can choose to make another bridge (counting the additional tooth that is ground down, this process then compromises four teeth, instead of three). Of course, as a consequence of elongating that bridge, more stress is placed on the teeth supporting that bridge. With time, the same thing that happened with the first bridge will happen with the second bridge. This creates kind of a domino effect, as the patient starts losing one tooth after another.

After a while, dentists encounter a limitation with bridges. A dentist can't typically create a bridge for a patient who has more than three teeth missing in the center of his or her mouth. In such cases, the dentist must craft a *removable partial denture*. Removable partial dentures are difficult to install because they actually sit on natural teeth. These devices are fitted with tiny clasps that hug the teeth to which they're attached, giving the denture stability. However, the clasps also put additional pressure on the patient's natural teeth, and over time the teeth will loosen. As a result, the patient ends up losing them prematurely. In other words, the patient starts with one lost tooth, and the dentist's solution compromises the function of three teeth. Then the patient has three teeth missing, which compromises the function of even more teeth. Using strong, healthy teeth to anchor these fixes in and then eventually sacrificing those teeth just does not make long-term sense for dentists or patients.

Here's the problem: At every stage of this traditional dentistry approach, all the dentist is doing is replacing the lost teeth. Nobody is actually looking at how the replacements are affecting the rest of the teeth. Because of that, the patient all too often finds him- or herself at the *edentulous* stage. At this stage, the patient has lost all of his or her natural teeth.

There are three main reasons why patients become fully toothless. The first reason is they have dental decay or dental cavities, a condition that causes the domino effect discussed above. The second reason patients lose their teeth is periodontal disease, also known as gum disease, which is also addressed above. Periodontal disease causes the foundation of an individual's teeth to loosen due to inflammation and bone loss around the teeth. (The loss of even a single tooth can play into this process, since shifting teeth can cause a domino effect of their own. Shifting teeth provide common sites for periodontal disease, since they create gaps in the gums that are difficult to clean). The third reason patients reach the fully toothless stage is because they simply do not want to deal with the pain of bad teeth any longer. They decide to remove all their teeth so that they can stop dealing with toothaches once and for all.

Today, thirty million Americans either have their full upper or full lower teeth missing, or have both arches missing, top and bottom. That number is staggering. It is equal to the entire population of Canada having no teeth.

Wearing dentures can present a number of challenges. The fact that dentures are removable prostheses means that people tend to drop them and break them—dentures are made of acrylic, so they break. And people frequently misplace their dentures. I've heard patients say, "I was in a restaurant. I took my teeth out to clean my mouth, but forgot to put them back in—and by the time I went back to look, my denture was gone." Then there is a scenario I have heard repeated many times: "I left them on the countertop, and my dog got them and chewed them." These are true stories.

Unfortunately, dentures present other challenges that are even more disconcerting. When someone wears a denture, his or her bite force is dramatically reduced. A person taking a regular bite is able to use two hundred pounds per square inch of pressure. With a denture, that force goes down to fifteen to fifty pounds of pressure per square inch. And that is only the initial decrease. After a patient wears a denture for fifteen years, bite pressure can amount to only six pounds per square inch. What does this mean? It means that the efficiency of chewing declines significantly. As I have already mentioned, one of the consequences of being unable to chew properly is an increase in gastrointestinal problems. (Heartburn, for example, is extremely common among denture wearers, probably because their difficulty in chewing means they swallow much of their food nearly whole). Of course, food selection itself becomes limited when chewing is a difficult proposition—denture-wearing patients' intake of healthy food, such as fruits and vegetables, is especially decreased.

The major problem presented by dentures, however, is the accelerated bone loss they cause in the jaw. To comprehend how this bone loss occurs, you must first understand that while a person's jawbone acts as the anchoring spot for his or her teeth, those teeth are actually what *keep* the jawbone in the mouth. The teeth's very presence, and the pressure they put on the bone as the person is chewing, stimulate the bone underneath and preserves its size and strength. The fact that pressure stimulates bone is the reason that doctors recommend people exercise to maintain skeletal bone mass. If you've ever had a broken arm or leg that was been placed in a cast, you've seen firsthand what happens when pressure isn't regularly applied: The limb that hasn't borne weight for weeks is visibly thinner when the cast comes off. True, some of that thinness is due to atrophied muscle. But some of it is due to loss of bone.

Once a dentist takes a patient's tooth away, there is nothing stimulating that bone any longer. Without that stimulation, the patient automatically loses 10 to 15 percent of the bone around the socket of that tooth (in both height and width) after just one year. I have models of jawbones in my office that I use to educate my patients about this subject. I can show them a model of a person's jawbone six months after teeth were removed and another model of the same bone ten years down the line. As anyone who sees these models can tell you, there is an extremely visible bone loss in both width and height. Once a patient loses teeth, his or her jawbone will begin to deteriorate.

Yet suppose you were to compare two patients who are missing all their teeth, one wearing a denture and the other totally *toothless* (i.e., not wearing anything). You would find the denture-wearing patient would show faster bone loss. That is because the denture itself has accelerated the patient's original bone loss, which was triggered by the absence of teeth. As the denture rests on top of the bone, it creates a different kind of pressure on the gum tissue, pressing against the gum and causing the tissue to become inflamed. In response to that inflammation, the body will actually make the bone disappear underneath that tissue. In such cases, patients deal with a double whammy: initial bone loss caused by disuse, since lack of natural tooth pressure isn't stimulating the area any more, and additional bone loss caused by this unnatural form of pressure.

Americans spend over two hundred million dollars each year on denture adhesive, a type of glue that helps keep dentures stable and in place against the gums. The amount of money spent annually to address the threat of denture-related embarrassment shows this is a major issue. Pretend, for a moment, you are wearing dentures. Initially, they feel okay. Of course, you had to deal with initial inflammation and soreness as your gums got accustomed to the pressure of dentures. You had to learn to speak all over again.[1] You had to learn

---

1   In my experience, about **88** percent of people who wear dentures report having speech problems. That is the same percentage reported in a

to eat all over again, and you had to learn to get used to the sensation of wearing a foreign object in your mouth. Yet, initially, your teeth feel stable, because your dentist made the denture to fit well against your tissue and bone—or, at least, what that tissue and bone looked like when your dentist originally made the denture.

Over a period of years, however, gradual bone loss will cause the denture to feel loose. I have patients who come in every two or three years, sometimes every year, because their dentures have gotten so loose that they are causing serious discomfort and even producing gum sores. In those cases, I either remake the denture or *reline* it (fill it with new acrylic to compensate for the bone that is been lost). Once again, these patients will have to endure a period of soreness as their gums adapt to the newly fitted dentures. Then things calm down, and they will feel okay for a while. However, the process of bone loss continues, and the cycle keeps going. Twenty years later, because of all the bone loss they have endured, these patients' dentures will probably be 400 percent taller. Small wonder, then, that in a study (the same one that identified speech problems in denture wearers), researchers found that more than 62 percent of people surveyed reported movement of their dentures within the mouth, while 63 percent reported discomfort. Clearly, some of these problems must have been severe: 16.5 percent of people surveyed in the study said they never wore their dentures at all.

To a dentist, it is easy to see how things can reach this point. Eventually a denture can become *free-floating*. In that case, there's simply not enough bone left to keep the denture in place. What's more, as bone is lost, the nerve that runs through it gets closer and

---

study conducted by my mentor, Dr. Misch. He also found that one-fourth of these people reported their problems were "difficult."

closer to the surface, until it eventually becomes exposed. Once that happens, the bone itself becomes extremely painful to the touch. At this point, patients who endure such pain will come to me, desperate for yet another fix. At this stage of bone loss, however, major reconstruction (which involves grafting of the bone) is the only solution that remains.

By now, you're probably thinking, as I once did, there must be a better way than heading down this disheartening road. There must be an alternative to going through the pain of bridges, partials, dentures, and bone loss. One alternative is to do simply nothing. In that case, the patient lives with tooth loss that gets progressively worse until he or she no longer has any teeth left. Truly, though, doing nothing is really not an option, given how it can destroy human health. Luckily, there is an option that preserves and even restores your health: The Dr. Bazzi Method™ of implant dentistry, a new procedure that makes up for the shortcomings of traditional dentistry.

CHAPTER
three

Dental Implants

A Modern-Day Miracle

Dental Implants

A Modern-Day Miracle

Despite the fact that modern implants are relatively new arrivals on the dental scene, implants themselves have a lengthy history. In Honduras, people have found "implanted" incisor teeth made from carved seashells in skulls dating back to AD 600. The Egyptians tried to do similar things with ivory, carving it into teeth shapes and trying to implant those shapes. In a way, implants aren't actually new; mankind has constantly tried to employ them to replace missing teeth for all the health reasons I have mentioned before.

Modern tooth implants, however, owe their origins to Dr. Per-Ingvar Branemark of Sweden, who created the titanium implants that are the standard today. Dr. Branemark began his experimental studies of titanium implants in 1952 and started putting them in patients in 1965, although he waited until 1977 to present his developments to the dental industry. The FDA recognized these implants in 1982. Today dentists place more than one million implants every year in the United States alone. As baby boomers age, this figure is going to grow. In fact, people anticipate that by 2025, dentists will be putting in between five and ten million implants a year.

As a dentist at the forefront of implant techniques, I've placed nearly one thousand implants myself. I routinely provide implants to elderly patients. As long as a person is in generally good health, age is no obstacle, I have found. Moreover, because these innovations restore lost chewing ability, improve appearance, end embarrassment, and give real self-confidence to patients who receive them, dental implants constitute a major breakthrough in both dental health and overall health. In fact, I consider them the most stable and economically far-sighted solution yet to the very real problem of missing teeth.

What Is an Implant and How Does It Work?

A dental implant is a biocompatible, man-made substitute for a missing tooth root, usually composed of a space-age titanium alloy. Think of it as the tooth's foundation: Just as the foundation of your home supports your house, an implant acts as the foundation for the tooth built on top of it. The type of implant most commonly used today—and the one I use in my own Dr. Bazzi Method™ of implant dentistry—is a cylinder fitted with screw-like threads. The dentist implants this cylinder into the bone of the jaw at the site where the lost tooth previously stood, and allows it to heal undisturbed. Over a period of several months, bone heals around the implant, locking it in like an anchor. At that point, the dentist inserts a prosthetic tooth into the implant.

The steps of the implant procedure itself are quite simple:

- First, if there is a damaged tooth, the dentist must ensure it is painlessly removed.

- Second, the dentist inserts the actual implant, that small threaded titanium post, into the patient's jawbone, under the gums. Local anesthesia and implementation of my signature sedation dentistry (which you will read more about in Chapter Six) make this a very comfortable process. In fact, the patient will not even remember the implant procedure.

- Third, once the implant itself is in place, the patient's body immediately begins to "bond" the titanium post into place with bone and tissue. This is a thorough healing process that may take anywhere from two to six months to complete. The patient's body does not reject the implant materials. Instead, the body ties them in with great strength, as if they were a natural part of the mouth. During the period in which this tying-in occurs, the patient will not walk around without teeth. That is a fear of many patients and a pet peeve of mine. Even in the most complicated cases, I can fashion a temporary denture. I always have a trick up my sleeve to ensure no one feels self-conscious while waiting for his or her new teeth to be placed permanently in position.

- Fourth, when the titanium implant has healed to the point where it is tied in securely, the dentist attaches a wider post to it by using a tiny screw. The dentist places a new tooth, one made of acrylic or porcelain, on this wider post, and cements it in using a resin that is so strong its bonding will virtually last forever.

- The patient now has a new tooth—and one that is indistinguishable from his or her other, natural teeth. The patient is the only one who knows it is man-made. And the implant is so comfortable that the patient soon forgets it is even there.

Implants represent a modern-day miracle for several reasons, but from the dentist's standpoint, a major one is this: They restore the original function of a lost tooth without negative impact to the rest of the patient's mouth. Implants work for one or two teeth, for several missing teeth, or even for the entire mouth, so they can take the place of bridges, partials, and dentures. However, they do not require sacrificing other teeth to anchor them, so that devastating domino effect of losing tooth after tooth does not happen. Moreover, since they allow patients to chew normally, using a natural degree of pressure, the bone loss experienced by people living with a missing tooth gap or with wearing dentures is effectively forestalled. The implants function like real teeth. They are truly the next best thing to your natural teeth.

As for the question of how long the implants last, anything that is put into the human body has its own medical success rate. The implants' success is measured in terms of five-year survival. (This means the implant remains in place, and is fully functional, for a period of five years). Nationally, about 92 percent of people's dental implants boast that five-year survival rate. My personal success rate for implants is higher: 95 to 97 percent of my patients make it past the five-year mark, which is extremely good. I can't give a 100-percent guarantee. There's nothing in medicine that is a 100-percent guarantee. However, my success rate means that for every 100 implants I have done, only three to five patients' implants have not made it to the five-year mark. (Most often the reason for this is a trauma that occurs well after I have placed the implants. For example, a car accident might dislodge them). Of the overwhelming majority of successful implants, most last far longer than just five years. I have patients in whom I placed implants more than a decade ago, and those implants are still functioning beautifully in their mouths. I am confident in saying that, typically, implants last a minimum of ten years. They will last much, much longer than dentures and have fewer associated problems.

A few caveats about implants: They do not decay, so cavities aren't a worry, but, as with other teeth, gum disease is. The gum surrounding the implants is the same as the gum tissue in the rest of the mouth, which means it suffers the same fate when subjected to neglect. If patients do not take proper care of the implants, if they do not clean them properly and go to the dentist on a regular basis, they can still get gum disease. Remember, gum disease can undermine bone, which means patients can still experience bone loss beneath and around the implants due to neglect. Basically, all the usual rules of dental hygiene hold for dental implants. People must brush. People must floss. People must use an antibacterial mouth rinse to make sure they kill germs in the mouth. People must treat implants as if they were real teeth, because, essentially, they are. Many patients do not even think about their implants as false teeth after a while. The implants feel like, act like, and should be treated like natural teeth.

As with any medical procedure, the implant procedure has associated possible risks and complications. A major risk is failed healing. If bone does not knit securely around the implant, the implant will fail because it isn't firmly anchored in place. For this reason, patients with health problems that can slow or impede healing aren't considered good candidates for implants (just as they aren't good candidates for other types of surgery). Conditions that can interfere with healing and make any surgery ill advised include uncontrolled diabetes, uncontrolled hypertension, hyperthyroidism, or mouth cancer.

Make no mistake; there's a difference between controlled and uncontrolled disease states here. For example, if a patient has controlled diabetes and is taking medications as advised, he or she can still receive implants. Often, there is a range of severity in which dentists can work. I'm always happy to consult with anyone in the hope that he or she can be helped. If a patient is high-risk, he or she may still be a candidate for implants. There are protocols that I follow and medications I can prescribe to mitigate some of those risks. I can place medical proteins underneath gum tissue during the implant surgery to increase the likelihood of successful healing, for example. If I can put enough positive forces into play and overcome the negatives associated with a patient's health challenges, and I have the patients' cooperation and understanding of the increased odds of implant failure, I will do my very best to improve their situation by trying to restore their teeth.

Smokers have an increased chance of complications from implant surgery, which means that patients who smoke will have a higher risk of losing an implant. This is because smoking decreases blood supply to the mouth. In this process, the patient and dentist rely on a good blood supply to bring cells to the mouth that help heal the tissue and create the strong bond between the titanium implant and the bone that will grow around it, anchoring it firmly in place. If a patient has less blood flow to the area, proper healing and bonding isn't ensured. If my patient is a smoker, I usually wait longer after doing the initial implants before I put the new post and tooth in place. (This allows for a longer healing period.) However, no dentist can determine exactly how much blood flow a patient has to a specific area, and if the blood flow is low, the implant may fail. It is not typical, but it does happen. Again, this information does not mean that smokers cannot, or should not, have dental implants done. It just means the patient and dentist need to do things a little differently to reduce the chances of having problems and increase the chances of achieving success.

There are also some anatomical risks to consider. Some patients come to me for implants after wearing dentures for thirty, forty, or even fifty years, and the longer they've been wearing dentures, the more pronounced their bone loss becomes. In some cases, the result is exposure of their *inferior alveolar nerve*, the pain-producing nerve I mentioned briefly before. This nerve is embedded within the lower jawbone, about a third of the way up from the bottom. As dentures accelerate bone loss from the upper surface of the jawbone, that buried nerve gets closer to the surface. If the nerve is too close, I can't put an implant there because, should the implant penetrate the nerve, the patient would suffer nerve damage that could lead to permanent numbness.

I have also seen patients whose bone loss is so severe their jawbones have become incredibly thin, like sheets of paper. To properly do an implant, a certain width and height of bone is required: the bone in which the implant is placed has to be solid, and that bone has to surround the implant from all sides. Neither the patient nor the dentist can have an implant sticking out of the bone. If the underlying structure isn't strong and thick enough, an implant will not work.

Still, even patients with paper-thin jawbones, or nerves that are fully or nearly exposed, can receive implants. The dentist just needs to create the bone in which the implants will be placed. To do this, I conduct bone grafting. Grafting involves taking bone from elsewhere in the body (another area of the mouth or, in very severe cases, the hip), shaping it into a section (or arch) matching the area that needs restoration, and connecting it to the *recipient bone*—the bone the patient still has—with a series of tiny screws. I then leave everything to heal for a period of six months. Once the grafted bone has merged with the recipient bone beneath it, I can go back and put the implants in.

One final note: Any patient who undergoes surgery deals with a risk of infection. Though the risk of infection associated with implants is minimal and only exists for the first week or so after the implantation, it is still a risk. To reduce the likelihood of infection, I make sure patients receive a course of oral antibiotics prior to and after their implant procedures.

Obviously, mitigating my patients' risks and complications associated with getting implants is a high priority for me. That is one reason why my success rates are so high. No matter how minor or remote a risk may seem, I fully inform my patients are of all risks. Is every patient who comes in going to get an infection? Hardly. It is very rare for a patient to get an infection, and the protocol I use makes such cases even rarer in my practice. Is every patient going to experience a nerve injury? No, because I am very careful in planning and making sure to stay away from the structures at which such injury could occur. Is every patient considered a high-risk candidate when it comes to implants? Absolutely not. However, if I have any indication that a patient is medically compromised, I will work with his or her physician so I can understand what needs to be done for that particular patient. I specialize in what I do, and I understand that other physicians specialize in what *they* do. If necessary, I consult with them to decrease the chances of complications for my patients.

CHAPTER
four

The Dr. Bazzi Method™
of Implant Dentistry

A State-of-the-Art Smile

The Dr. Bazzi Method™ of Implant Dentistry

A State-of-the-Art Smile

By now, you have learned the basics about implant dentistry. I hope too you have learned a bit about me. I have shared my passion for the implant process as a superior, state-of-the art solution to tooth loss and the health problems associated with it. I have described my expertise as a surgeon who has done implants for a decade and a half. I have explained my higher-than-average success rate in performing more than a thousand implant procedures. However, I developed my method—the Dr. Bazzi Method™ of implant dentistry—from more than just years of high-level training and experience. In a very real way, I developed it from the heart.

In my practice, my talented team of professionals and I do not just care for our patients. We care about them. They are people who matter a great deal to me, and they matter to my team. I spend a great deal of time with my patients, and I understand that they spend a great deal of time with me. I deeply appreciate their commitment to improving their oral health and overall health. As we work together, I get to know them very well, so well that they become a part of my extended family. At work, patients come up and give me hugs all the time, saying, "This is the best thing I have ever done in my life." That is the ultimate reward of the work I do. It is also why I think of my practice model as an ever-evolving system of continuous care. At my practice, my relationship with a patient may start with one consultation or one implant surgery. However, the Dr. Bazzi Method™ of implant dentistry is more than consultations, diagnoses, and installing implants. You might recall my earlier statement that if I give a patient implants, that patient is with me for life. Once again, that is exactly how I feel. I am there for my patients from the first appointment on, working with them to solve their tooth problems. After the problems they have today are solved, I will be there for them if they need me in the future.

Historically, the dental profession has not had the best reputation when it comes to caring. Moreover, fear of pain remains an obstacle for many individuals. What I have found is that people are people. Like me, they want to be treated with respect, kindness, and gentleness, and when they are treated in this spirit, they can overcome obstacles such as fear and mistrust. I have gone outside my profession to learn this, and I practice it in my personal life. I also owe my own mother an enormous debt of gratitude for this knowledge. She taught me to treat others with the same kindness and consideration that I wanted them to show to me. Yes, I treat dental problems. But I also treat people, people about whom I care a great deal.

I also understand that no two people are alike. Each one of my patients has a different set of health concerns and conditions, anatomical variations, life circumstances, and priorities. All of these factors play into what constitutes the best care for each individual. Because of this distinctiveness, I customize each patient's treatment plan, developing unique solutions for each on a highly individualized basis. The Dr. Bazzi Method™ of implant dentistry is not a cookie-cutter approach. Over my years of experience, I have learned there is no such thing as a textbook case. I dedicate myself to providing carefully customized care and treatment plans for every patient, and to carrying out these plans in ways targeted to each one's complex set of personal needs.

My practice also offers patients another type of ever-evolving care, in that the knowledge I bring to every aspect of treatment is constantly improving. I had the benefits of an outstanding education in dental school, followed by the privilege of working with one of the most renowned and respected experts in implant dentistry. But I did not stop there; I continue to expand my knowledge and skills, and I stay up to date with new advancements and techniques. I attend seminars and take courses regularly. I read the latest journals in my field almost every day. I keep up with everything that is going on in the field of dentistry in general and in implant dentistry in particular.

The Dr. Bazzi Method™ of implant dentistry is one of exacting standards—namely, the standards I set for myself. I am a perfection-ist by nature. If there is something I do not like, I fix it. Often, patients will look at their teeth before I am completely done with their treatment and say, "Oh, this looks great!" Yet if I find there is something that could look a tad better, I do it. I am my own worst critic. Every patient's final results must meet the high standards I set for my practice and for myself. I will go above and beyond to ensure this happens.

For example, sometimes I am not 100 percent happy with a crown that the laboratory technicians have fabricated on my behalf, so I send it back to them for modifications. If I am doing a particu-larly complicated case, I have the laboratory technician in my office should I need him. I then get the technician's undivided attention.

He knows exactly what I need for the patient because he is there too, looking at the patient himself. You do not get that kind of benefit everywhere. Not every dentist has that kind of relationship with their laboratory that enables getting the technician to the patient's side if needed. I have established that kind of relationship, and I am proud of doing so, since it is a superior arrangement for the patient.

I am also meticulous in engineering the teeth so the top and bottom rows meet each other properly. This ensures that the patient can chew and grind food efficiently. You may recall that the mouth is the beginning of the digestive system. Chewing is the key first step in the digestive process. It breaks down food into small pieces that can then be optimally digested. Chewing also increases production of saliva, which contains enzymes that start to digest food even before swallowing. Efficient chewing makes the entire digestive process go much more smoothly. Thus, gastrointestinal problems are either eliminated or significantly diminished as one happy consequence of the Dr. Bazzi Method™.

Of course, another consequence of my complete refusal to compromise on the level of care I administer to my patients, and the final results they get, is an absolutely beautiful smile. I want my patients to feel renewed confidence. I want to see the difference in their appearance, their attitudes, and the quality of their lives that I know the Dr. Bazzi Method™ of implant dentistry can make. I also want to ensure that if one of my patients were to move out of town and visit another dentist, that dentist would look in his or her mouth and say, "Wow! Who did this for you?" And that patient, feeling confident and happy, would proudly say, "I met this dental implantologist in Michigan, and…"

As a prospective patient, not a dentist, you will not get the chance to hear from these patients. However, you can hear from patients of mine. Many of them are so happy with their implants that they have agreed to share their experience with others who are interested in becoming patients. Many people have written to me to about the differences the Dr. Bazzi Method™ of implant dentistry has made in their lives. Here's a small sampling of such testimonials:

My natural teeth had been a source of embarrassment and pain for many years. The embarrassment was difficult enough to deal with, but the pain was excruciating at times.

I will never forget waking up and discovering that several of the crowns in the front were loose. My biggest fear was having my teeth fall out while I was talking. I carried a mirror in my purse so I could check my teeth several times a day and make sure they were all there. I couldn't smile as much as I wanted to, since I was afraid people would see my teeth—or lack of teeth.

At Dr. Bazzi's office, I had many questions and the team answered all of them completely. We scheduled the surgery, and after years of avoidance I was actually looking forward to starting the process. I was given medication before and after the surgery so I felt ready to deal with the pain. After my surgery, I took the pain medication as prescribed and then slept for several hours. Upon waking, I had no pain. I immediately ran to the mirror and was completely surprised. My healing teeth looked great, and I was ready to face the world with a smile.

My happiness this past year has increased a hundredfold, since years' worth of stress have been lifted from my life. I have also started appearing in family photos after a thirty-year absence. That will be a mystery to future generations when they review family albums!

My story would not be complete without giving complete credit and thanks to Dr. Bazzi. From my initial phone call last year to this point, I have experienced quality care from all members of his team at each and every appointment. I will forever be grateful for finding Dr. Bazzi and entrusting my dental needs to his care. His expertise, professionalism, and sense of humor have taken me from hopelessness to happiness over the past year.

—Barbara, implant and sedation dentistry patient

When I, with five hopeless teeth, first saw my dentist, I was certain there would be no option other than dentures. The next best thing had seemed to be extensive bridgework. I was pleased and enthusiastic to learn of the possibility of implants.

The best help came from Dr. Bazzi's careful explanation of the future work. At the time, I found it all hard to imagine. However, as the work progressed it was systematic and obvious. One of the most interesting parts of the adventure was seeing the molds of my jaw with all the new work in place.

Now I have had my well used and admired implants for seven years. I am now seventy-five years old and have had diabetes for twenty years, so Dr. Bazzi needed an okay from my MD before the procedure. All went well during and after the procedure. I observed that Dr. Bazzi has fine dental skills and people skills. Besides these qualities, he has the artistic skills of Michelangelo and the craftsmanship of Paul Revere.

I am proud and pleased to recommend Dr. Bazzi's work, and the adventure in general, to anyone.

— Ruth, implant and sedation dentistry patient

Approximately two and a half years ago, I had new dentures made. For two years, I struggled to eat! I got sores from the plates rubbing on my gums, which made attempting to chew painful. After numerous adjustments, including being fitted for and purchasing a liner, I continued having the problem. My former dentist informed me that I would probably have to replace the liner twice a year at the cost of $500 each time. I was very disappointed. That was when I saw Dr. Bazzi's ad and set up a consultation appointment. He explained my options, what to expect with the surgery, and what would happen after surgery.

Everything went exactly as I was told it would, and I had no pain to speak of. The quality of my life has improved greatly. I can now sit down to a meal and not have to worry about improperly fitting dentures. I would highly recommend Dr. Bazzi and his staff for their professionalism.

—Roy, implant and sedation dentistry patient

Due to many years of not having dental insurance and not doing the best job at oral care, my teeth had become embarrassing to me. The front teeth overlapped, some were missing, and I was always having some sort of abscess or other oral issue.

I decided to get proactive about my dental health and looked for a dentist who could provide solutions to my problems. I came to Dr. Bazzi for a consultation. He offered it for free, and it was very thorough. Dr. Bazzi made me feel comfortable. I could feel his compassion, and I knew I could trust him to take care of me.

Dr. Bazzi proposed the solution of fitting me with implanted teeth. The process started with the extraction of my poorest teeth (leaving me with seven of my own natural teeth). Dr. Bazzi immediately fitted me with a denture to use while my mouth healed. The drugs used for this first procedure were completely effective, and I was back at work in four days. At this stage, it was very nice to have a mouth full of teeth that would actually grind and chew food, and I appreciated the fact that I could smile without embarrassment.

The next steps were equally pain-free; Dr. Bazzi and his staff always provided me with the best care and treatment. Now that my implant dental work is complete, I will continue to see Dr. Bazzi and his team for regular dental care.

—Don, implant and sedation dentistry patient

I am also proud to say that many other professionals in the field of dentistry—including my mentor, Dr. Misch—recommend my work without reservation. Some of their comments include the following:

Dr. Nader Bazzi was one of my two externs [interns] in the discipline of implant prosthodontics and implant dentistry. I directly observed his abilities to communicate with patients and professionals and provide implant surgery and prosthetics.

Dr. Bazzi has excellent abilities in the field of implant dentistry. He also has a passion for the delivery of proper care. His experience over the years has demonstrated a care for patients' needs. As a result, I have often asked Dr. Bazzi to treat my patients when I have been out of town or on vacation.

In summary, Dr. Bazzi possesses strong credentials that will prove to be an asset to our dental community. I strongly, and with complete confidence, recommend him for your treatment.

—Carl E. Misch, DDS, MDS, Misch Implant Institute

Dr. Nader Bazzi is Canton's premier implant dentist. In fact, he is one of the best in the entire Detroit region. Dr. Bazzi has trained with the top dentists in the profession worldwide. He will do a great job of giving you comfortable chewing and a smile that you will be proud to share. You are quite privileged to have such a skilled clinician available to you. He can handle the most complicated situations and is an expert at helping even those most hopeless patients. Let Dr. Bazzi help you. You will be glad you did.

—Dr. James McAnally, implant and sedation dentistry clinician, consultant, and dental author

Dr. Bazzi is the most caring and dedicated dentist. He has shown himself be both a great dentist and a master craftsman in his profession. His attention to detail is second to none, allowing him to provide the absolute best dentistry for everyone he treats. Dr. Bazzi has traveled extensively throughout the world to train with the best in implant dentistry. I can highly recommend Dr. Bazzi.

—Dr. Davis Kagan, DDS

CHAPTER
five

The Patients Who Can Benefit
from the Dr. Bazzi Method™

The Patients Who Can Benefit from the Dr. Bazzi Method™

My ideal patient is one who has a problem, is aware of it, and wants and needs to have that problem taken care of as soon as possible. This ideal is not terribly restrictive. I tackle a wide range of problems daily. That is one thing that makes it easy for me to enjoy doing what I do. People suffer needlessly from so many dental concerns. It is a constant thrill for me to witness the transformations that occur when those concerns are resolved. I love nothing more than having people tell me what they dislike about their teeth, or what they worry about regarding their dental care experience, and then figuring out solutions that leave those people happier and healthier. In fact, that is probably why I love implants so much: They provide such a terrific solution. Implants allow me to provide what I feel is the absolute best of today's dentistry, and, in doing so, to give patients back full teeth functionality, a beautiful smile, and the psychological wholeness that goes along with those things.

Age is absolutely not a limiting factor when it comes to candidacy for implants. This allows me to treat a wide range of patients. My team and I do implants on patients as young as sixteen (women) and eighteen (men).[2] We also do implants on patients who are in their eighties and nineties. As I noted previously, no patient is too old for us to perform the procedure—provided the patient is in good health, of course.

However, there are a few people for whom implant surgery is not the right choice. I have already described several medical conditions that can make people inappropriate candidates for implants. My team and I do not perform implants on pregnant women, simply because scientists have not conducted research on implants and pregnancy. Other medical issues can also preclude a patient from getting implants. I can work with these people on an individual basis, provided I receive their physician's assurance that doing the procedure will not harm them (if, for example, someone was currently undergoing chemo or radiation treatment in the mouth).

In addition, I sometimes encounter patients who have unrealistic expectations about how quickly their treatment can be accomplished or how cheaply it can be done. Other times, patients truly cannot, or will not, take regular care of their mouths. In such cases, implants are destined to fail, and they will not be worth the initial expense and effort. When I encounter patients for whom implants do not make a viable option, I recommend alternatives that will fit their needs.

---

2   The age difference between men and women is due to the fact that men's bones, including their jawbones, take longer to mature than women's. The crown I use over the implant is designed to match the patient's other teeth. If the dentist puts in an implant while the patient is still growing, the implant tooth will eventually look shorter than the adjacent teeth. There is, unfortunately, no reliable way to allow for continuing growth.

Finally, implant dentistry is an elective procedure that must not be performed when a patient is going through any life-changing events. It has to be a proper fit for the patient's life situation.

However, aside from these few exceptions, almost anyone can benefit from this fabulous method. In fact, odds are *you* fit into one (if not more!) of the excellent-candidate categories below:

- People who want to preserve their remaining teeth when a tooth is unexpectedly lost or broken. Typically, these people have taken good care of their teeth and just happen to have had a misfortune with one tooth. They value the state of their mouths and understand the need to replace that tooth immediately so their other teeth don't shift. These patients, who are committed to a high level of dental health, are patients I adore. They understand the importance of their oral health and its implications for their general health. I am proud to have these people as members of my patient family.

- People who are frustrated by, or just plain tired of, dealing with the practical problems and pain associated with partial or full dentures. They are sick of the gooey denture adhesive. They are sick of sore gums and the embarrassment they suffer when their teeth literally fall out in public. I have heard far too many horror stories from patients who were in public situations and had their dentures fall out in front of friends or colleagues. I call this Murphy's law of denture movement: Dentures that float around in the mouth will become displaced at the worst possible times. Often the bone loss caused by wearing dentures is the culprit behind these embarrassments. The bone loss becomes so extensive that there is nothing for the dentures to secure themselves against. At this point, even denture adhesives will not work, or they will work for a half-hour to forty-five minutes at most. When adhesives stop working, Murphy's law of denture movement rules. This leads to extremely humiliating experiences, and such experiences are often what lead people, in turn, to seek my services.

- People who have replacement bridges they really do not like. Patients who already have bridges often dislike the way the foreign bridge feels in their mouths, and/or they dislike not being able to floss between their teeth. They ask me to remove the bridge, put an implant in the center of the problem area, and put individual crowns over their teeth.

- People who do not want removable teeth at all. I have had some patients who were extremely fearful of having removable teeth in their mouths. Some even had nightmares when they first heard about the prospect of dentures, and their fear led them to seek me out.

- People in whom progressive bone loss is causing a loss of support for the face and changing their appearance for the worse. Again, when people lose teeth, bone loss is sure to follow. As a consequence, the cheeks and lips start to crease more, causing more wrinkles. Dental implants put teeth where they need to be—supporting the lips and cheeks, thereby giving a youthful fullness back to the face. In fact, implants have been shown to shave ten to fifteen years off a person's appearance.

- People who have missing teeth, or are about to lose teeth, due to decay or fracture. Patients who avoid seeing a dentist can actually live unknowingly with cavities and decay for years. When they finally do seek dental care, they find out that at least one of their teeth is beyond repair because decay has reached deep down into the bone.

- People who have significant gum disease. As you may already know, gum disease destroys the foundation of bone around the teeth. When all the teeth are affected, the person has so much bone loss that his or her teeth become loose. There is nothing a dentist can do at this stage.[3]

- People who have just "had it" with their teeth. These patients have suffered a series of constant tooth problems and toothaches. They have become entirely fed up. They typically have a "mouthful" of problems that seem to get worse and worse. Rather than risk dealing with yet another event, they want a permanent fix. The reasons for their oral health problems may vary from bad habits to

---

3   Many people are not aware of this, but gum disease is transmittable. That means that if you are kissing your partner or sharing a plate of food with your child, the bacteria get transferred from one person to another. If you have gum disease, you have to take care of your problem so that you do not pass on the problem to your loved ones.

bad genes to bad luck. The reasons do not matter. At my practice, we never judge patients for what has happened in their mouths or in their lives. What we do, instead, is give them a solution. For example, I will remove all of a person's teeth, top and bottom, and replace them with a full set of implants. At one time, the only option for these patients was to get full dentures (which meant they would eventually fall prey to bone loss, premature aging, potential embarrassment, and more pain.) Today, because of implants, we dentists are able to take bad teeth out and put fully functional, good teeth in.

- People who want to prevent the domino effect of sacrificing more and more teeth, and losing underlying bone, which happens when dentists use traditional methods to replace one tooth that cannot be saved. Think back to the discussion of how mother nature handles a missing tooth: Bone loss occurs at the site. Then, shifting and hypereruption occur in other teeth. Think back to the discussion of what happens when dentists use bridges to replace lost teeth: The dentist grinds down the surrounding teeth on either side and fits them with crowns that will eventually give under pressure. This situation can progress to the point where the patient starts looking at dentures or a full set of implants. However, the speedy replacement of a lost tooth with an implant can arrest such cycles. If I find a patient's tooth is hopeless, for whatever reason, I can remove the tooth, do a small amount of bone grafting in the socket (so the surrounding bone does not shrink), let the area heal for three months, and then go back and put in an implant.

Receiving such immediate attention is the best scenario for the patient.

- People who have suffered an accident that has affected their teeth, and who want to regain their original tooth functionality and appearance. These are all my auto or bike-accident patients whose teeth have been knocked out, as well as all my teenage friends who fell out of a tree and dislodged a front tooth that couldn't be saved.

- People whose teeth are perfect—except for one or two, that is. These patients would like to have a perfect smile. In their cases, my team and I remove the few crooked teeth and replace them with implants in a more desirable position. If a patient is only concerned about one or two teeth, using implants can help him or her achieve smile perfection in as little as three months. Contrast this process to that of orthodontics, which can take about two years.

- People who are disappointed by earlier attempts to fix their teeth. These patients have had a bad experience and are looking for a makeover. They are considering dental implants to take care of disappointments caused by the traditional dentistry methods they have had in the past.

- People who want to enjoy their golden years. When it is time to retire, people want to be able to socialize with colleagues, friends, and family. Much of that socializing involves food. If someone has poor oral health or is missing teeth, he or she will be less likely to enjoy that quality of life. I see this all the time. These patients arrive at our clinic miserable and depressed. As soon as we take care of them and give them proper teeth, their entire lives turn around. They become much happier and enjoy a much higher quality of life.

- People who are finally ready to have major dental work done. These patients have not been to a dentist in the past twenty or thirty years. Perhaps it is the wisdom that comes with age, or the fact that they have tired of listening to a nagging mental voice telling them they know better than to neglect their situation. Something finally motivates these people to gather their courage and come to my team for a consultation. I find working with these patients highly rewarding. My team and I are able to allay their fears quickly, and, just as quickly, these patients come to recognize the high level of service we provide. They start looking forward to getting their implants done. They realize the attention to their teeth is long overdue. Taking care of things becomes an enormous relief.

- People who want cutting-edge technology and state-of-the-art technique. These people include tech-savvy patients and computer engineers who only want the best treatment available. In today's world, this treatment is the best. The procedure itself is extremely quick, which is something else that makes these patients adore what my team does. They love the fact that they do not have to take too much time off from work because of this procedure.

- People who deserve the best dentistry can offer for solving the wide range of problems associated with missing teeth. Dental implants are currently the best solution for restoring lost teeth, and they are far superior to older replacement methods. In the future, in 2050 and beyond, dental professionals hope to be able to implant cells in the bone so a tooth could grow out of the gum tissue, just like a flower would. However, this is dependent upon the development of genetic engineering. Until then, dental implants stand ready to solve problems now.

- People who want to recapture their smiles' youthful appearance through a combination of dental implants and veneers. These patients may have gaps between their teeth or crooked teeth. They may have had a lot of dental work that is showing its age—work done at a time when techniques did not give the aesthetically pleasing results that implants give today. These patients always yearn for a youthful-looking smile. My team and I grant this wish by using a combination of dental implants (on any teeth that need to be replaced) and veneers (on natural, yet time-worn or yellowed teeth).

- People who want to address their current dental concerns and, in doing so, prevent future problems. To give just one example of this, I want to look at bone loss again. Years ago, if a patient had a tooth removed, no dentist would mention the fact that the person was going to suffer bone loss once that tooth came out. Part of the informed consent process I undertake with my patients includes educating them about the long-term consequences of any treatment they are considering. I educate patients about the bone loss that can occur if even one tooth is pulled and not replaced immediately. Because that bone loss begins immediately, I encourage patients who need implants to have them done right away. My patients are not dentists. They cannot be expected to understand the process of bone loss and its consequences until a dentist explains it to them. It is critical that I educate them so they do understand—for the sake of their long-term health.

- People who see the common sense of applying the Dr. Bazzi Method™ of implant dentistry to their personal situations. These patients have examined the advantages of implants themselves, as well as the time-tested, successful techniques I have developed within my practice, and concluded that the Dr. Bazzi Method™ of implant dentistry is an intelligent choice.

CHAPTER
six

Getting Your Implants

A New Smile in One Day!

Getting Your Implants

A New Smile in One Day!

I staunchly believe that an informed, educated patient makes the best decisions. With this belief in mind, my patients receive all the information they need to make those best decisions. I begin to educate prospective patients before they walk into my office. Once I receive a referral, I mail the patient information about me, my training and qualifications, my treatment philosophy, my practice and our services, and general guidelines about associated costs. This information helps people prepare for their initial free consultation with me.

The Initial Consultation

The initial consultation is a free visit that typically takes fifteen to thirty minutes. In that very brief time, it serves a number of vital purposes. For one thing, it gives people a chance to see my practice's aesthetics, which is extremely important to me. People cannot learn how good my work is just by reading about it. They cannot realize how much my team and I care simply by being told. However, when they see my office, they get firsthand information about how clean and pleasing to the eye everything is. They get to meet my wonderful staff and view the state-of-the-art equipment we have in place. That is important in conveying my commitment to quality and in making people feel comfortable—putting them at ease. Many of my patients will comment, "You know, I love your office. I love how clean it is and how everybody on your team is so pleasant and nice." I love it when they say things like that. I consider everything when it comes to providing my patients with a positive experience, and a welcoming, yet professional, environment is part of that experience.

This consultation is a valuable first opportunity for my team and me to hear about a patient's concerns and get a sense of his or her expectations. It is also a valuable opportunity for the patient to get to know us. From the beginning of each relationship, I want patients to be able to speak freely with me and know that I do not prejudge them in any fashion. Some have not gone to a dentist in ten, fifteen, or twenty or more years, and they can experience shame and disgust over the state of their oral health. I want to make sure that they are not coming in to an environment where someone would ever say, "Hey, why did you do this to yourself?" My team and I do not know the circumstances people have encountered in their lives. We do not know what kind of problems they have had. We do not want to judge people. We want to put them at ease.

During the first part of each consultation, my team and I give patients an overview of what is possible in implant dentistry. We then let the patients talk, so we can learn about what they want. My highly qualified dental assistants drive most of these exchanges. They will ask the patients general questions: What brings you here? What is your main concern? What are you hoping to get from treatment? Can you tell us a little about your past experiences with dentists? Then, my team members will listen. That is vitally important. In fact, listening to the patient is more important than I can convey. Once my team members have listened to and learned about each patient's concerns and needs, they will briefly educate him or her about what's possible with implant dentistry. Using medical models of the jaws and teeth, they will explain the technology and the techniques, applying them to the patient's individualized situation and unique history.

Following this portion of the visit, one of my dental assistants will meet with me and give me a synopsis about the patient, sharing what he or she has learned from the interaction. I will then introduce myself to the patient, talk with and listen to him or her. During this exchange I will not share specifics about the patient's upcoming treatment for two valid reasons: First, I do not yet know enough about the patient's teeth to give specifics. Second, I want to get a sense of what the patient wants and expects, so I can make sure I am able to meet—and beat—those expectations.

Some patients have unrealistic expectations. They will come in for their first consultations in April and want everything done by the end of May. They will want all their work done for an unrealistic cost or want to negotiate with me for only what their insurance will pay. For reasons you already understand (and others you will soon understand), some of these expectations are not realistic. Proper treatment and complete healing take time. This process cannot be rushed. Costs of treatment will extend beyond insurance coverage, which is typically poor. Most people understand these things, but I still encounter patients who do not, especially those who have not sought dental services in years. If the patient and I have a gap in our expectations about such things, the initial consultation allows us to discuss them. The consultation allows us to get on the same page. However, I do not cut corners in delivering care.

If a patient likes us and feels comfortable with us—and I am proud to say the overwhelming majority do—then we go to the next step, which is scheduling the diagnostic appointment.

The Diagnostic Appointment

At this visit, the patient comes into our office and we make him or her comfortable in one of our examining rooms. We then gather medical data on the state of the patient's mouth and teeth. This can involve a variety of steps: We take a panoramic X-ray of the entire mouth and may take smaller X-rays of specific sites as needed. We take pictures of the upper and lower jaw. We take pictures of the patient's smile, as well as any diseased teeth or gum problems. We also make models of the upper and lower jaw (these are called *study models*, since they are for me to study after the patient leaves).

I then do a thorough examination of the patient's gums, measuring them and determining their condition. I also do a complete visual examination of the teeth and bones. I check the bone's angle, quantity, and quality. I assess the jaw relations: how the upper and lower jaws meet. I assess the temporomandibular joints and ensure they have no preexisting problems. All of this is part of the data gathering that constitutes the diagnostic appointment.

One thing worth noting: None of this hurts a bit. My team and I make sure every part of the process is comfortable. For example, some patients I see have loose teeth, a condition usually caused by gum disease (eventually, periodontal disease reaches the bone level and eats away at the bone, making the teeth loose). These patients can experience fear and anxiety over the impressions we take of their teeth to make our study models. They ask questions like, "Will my teeth come out when you take the impressions?" That is a legitimate question, though I must say it is only a concern for about one in every twenty or so patients. However, we make sure it does not happen, and we do so in a very simple way: We place Vaseline on the teeth to make them slippery, so they do not stick to the material we use when taking the impressions.

At the end of the data-gathering process, we schedule a third visit for about a week later. This is the treatment presentation appointment.

The Treatment Presentation

During this appointment, the patient meets with me in my office consultation room. My treatment coordinator will also be there, listening carefully during the meeting. That way, if the patient has any questions after I leave the room, the treatment coordinator can properly address them. I also strongly suggest that someone close to the patient (a good friend or family member) attend this meeting as well. I want my patients to have support every step of the way. Once they leave the office, I want them to be able to talk to someone close to them, someone who has also listened to everything that I had to say and can provide support in making a good decision. The traditional method of meeting with patients—alone—means the patients have to go home and show their report and its findings to a spouse, family member, or friend. However, those parties will not have the direct opportunity to ask questions of me. I prefer to have my patient's supportive people right there, so if they have any questions, I can answer them right away.

By the time we sit down for the treatment presentation, I will have prepared a comprehensive ten- to twenty-page report based upon all the previously gathered information. The report, which covers all my findings, includes pictures and X-rays of the mouth, the bite, and the smile. It clearly identifies what the patient's major concerns are. The report also gives my findings and recommendations for treatment. I go through the report in an absolutely nonjudgmental way, making sure my patients are at ease. I always tell them, "Please stop me if you have any questions. I am here to educate both of us on what is going on with you." I do not go over what happened in the patients' past. That does not matter. Together, the patient and I look at the present and move forward toward the future. After we have gone over the findings, I present my treatment recommendations: the solutions that will return the patient's mouth to a healthy state.

In presenting these solutions, I address the consequences of *not* treating the mouth (by this point in the process, most patients are already aware their situation is only going to worsen if they do nothing). I then give three treatment options: one good, one better, and one that I consider the best. I discuss each of these recommendations fully, covering the advantages and disadvantages in terms of what each will involve and how they will affect the patient's daily life. Then, I let the patient choose the one that he or she feels is right.

Obviously, I develop each treatment option according to the respective patient's unique needs—I cannot stress enough that no two patients are alike. However, in general, the options for extensive tooth replacement fall into three categories:

- The Platinum Standard: In what I consider a superior option, I fix all of the patient's prosthetic teeth in place. The teeth do not come out. Typically, I will place a total of six to eight implants in the mouth and then design the teeth, which the lab technicians will fashion. The teeth themselves have a porcelain exterior, which lends a more natural appearance to the end result. The porcelain used in the lab is also glazed, which gives each tooth a smooth finish that does not allow bacteria or food particles to stick to it easily. Therefore, patients who receive porcelain teeth will encounter much less staining than they would with acrylic teeth.

The lab technicians use gold to make the interior of the teeth. People do not see the gold, because it is on the inside, but that is what connects the teeth together. In the lab, the technicians fuse the porcelain exterior onto the gold interior. The tooth comes back to me in a single piece that I place in the upper or lower arch of the patient's mouth. I then cement this prosthesis in place over the implants. This option looks the most natural. In fact, to the patient, it appears identical to the natural teeth. The materials I use make this the strongest and longest-lasting option. It also requires less maintenance than the other two options.

- The Gold Standard: This process is similar to the treatment described above in that the teeth are nonremovable. I cement them in place in the patient's mouth over six to eight implants. The prefabricated teeth are usually made out of acrylic, but the patient can also select prefabricated porcelain teeth.

No matter what the choice, I fuse these teeth over a metal alloy that adds inner support to the teeth (without that, they would break very easily). I then cement the resulting arch over the implants, which I have already put in place. I should note here that my team and I can be flexible with many specifics in these general categories. For example, sometimes I have patients who want their teeth to look more natural, but they cannot afford to go the Platinum route. My team and I can give them porcelain teeth that I imbed into the acrylic framework (I still place the metal alloy underneath this framework, in order to keep the teeth stronger). In this and other ways, we will work with the patient's needs and wants.

- The Silver Standard: This option is the closest to conventional full dentures. While bulkier than the Gold or Platinum treatments, it is still less bulky than traditional dentures are. Typically, during this process I put in four to six implants, and I connect the implants with a bar. I then make the rest of the teeth fit over the bar. This marks a major improvement over conventional dentures, since the palate or roof of the mouth is not covered.

  In this scenario, I permanently fix the implants and the bar in place, while ensuring the teeth fitting over them are removable. Patients can take these teeth out for cleaning and hygiene purposes (I recommend removing and cleaning them on the same schedule one would use for dentures, which includes cleaning after every meal). Then, they simply snap back the teeth on to the bar connected to those implants. This means the teeth are locked firmly in place, which is another advantage over conventional dentures, since those often move around inside the mouth.

Comparison of Dental Implant Options Available with Dr. Bazzi Method Modern Dental Implants

(All photos from the perspective of looking up at the palate.)

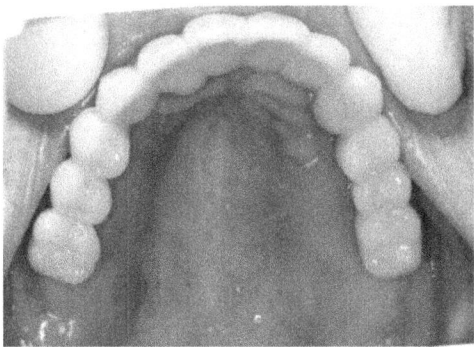

The Platinum Standard: nonremovable porcelain implant teeth no plastic, no gagging, feels and looks like natural teeth

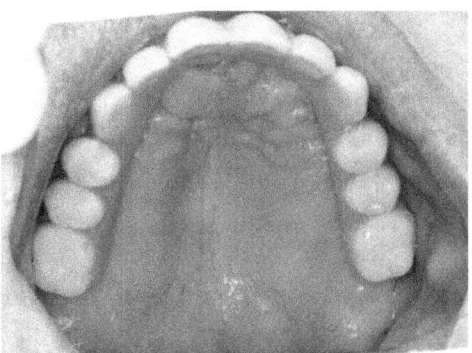

The Gold Standard: nonremovable porcelain/acrylic implant teeth 95 percent less plastic than a denture; feel and look like natural teeth

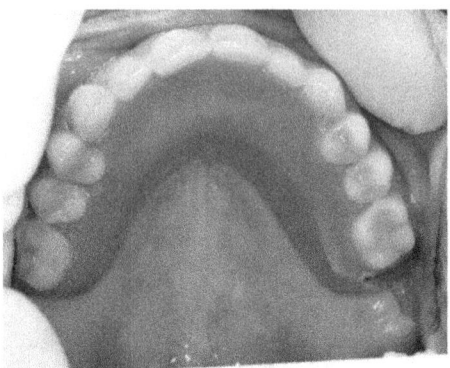

The Silver Standard: removable porcelain/acrylic implant teeth, feel almost like natural teeth and look like natural teeth

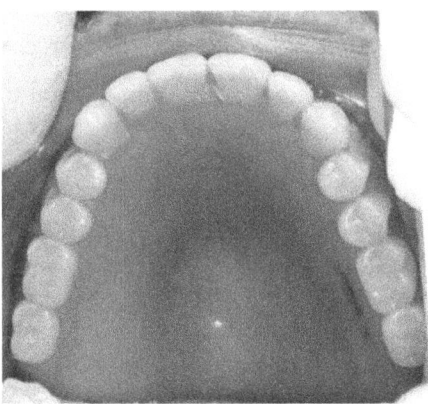

The Eighteenth-Century Standard, a Denture: bulky, gags, interferes with taste, unhygienic, denture goop-glue required

As you might imagine, the Platinum, Gold, and Silver options also differ in cost: Platinum is the most expensive and Silver the cheapest. Even so, about 95 percent of my patients opt for Platinum. About 2 or 3 percent choose Gold, and about the same number choose Silver.

You may have noticed that I mentioned easier maintenance as a distinct advantage. Maintenance is vital for any implant. I devote special attention to my treatment presentations. Some patients like to have the least amount of maintenance possible. Others do not mind a little extra work in taking care of their mouths. I always tailor the different options I present to how I think the patient will do in terms of maintenance. Ultimately, whichever option the patient selects, I have to make sure he or she is able to maintain it satisfactorily. Otherwise, no matter what treatment the patient selects (and no matter how good the dentist is who does it), that treatment will end up failing. I want success for all my patients, so I make sure to stress the importance of maintenance.

Some patients need help with financing the treatment they decide to pursue. This is where my treatment coordinator takes over. She will discuss a variety of financing strategies with the patient. (I cover these more fully in Chapter Nine). She will also work with the patient to put preliminary financing programs in place.

By this point, many patients feel comfortable enough to schedule the treatment itself. Others may be undecided, so I set a follow-up appointment in another week's time. This gives the patients the opportunity to digest everything we've presented and come back to us with further questions. Once they are comfortable with the treatment they choose, we can then schedule the implant procedure.

The Implant Procedure: A Smile in One Day

A Smile in One Day is a revolutionary process. It is something that I created. As recently as five or ten years ago it was not possible to perform this process. When my colleagues and I were doing implant dentistry, we would have to do the different steps in stages and allow each patient a healing period. A patient would come in with no teeth, but not receive their teeth and be completely finished with the healing process until about two years later.

Today the Dr. Bazzi Method™ of implant dentistry significantly cuts down on the time it takes to get a new smile. For instance, I had a patient come in recently with a full mouth of teeth that were broken down and could not be saved. Traditionally, a dentist would have taken out the teeth, given the patient a denture, and let the mouth heal for a period of six months. After that, the patient would return for another visit so the dentist could rebuild the bone by grafting it. The dentist would have to let *that* heal for another four to six months before putting the implants in. Then, the dentist would have to let the implants heal for a period of six months, before adding the teeth. In this recent patient's scenario, however, my team and I removed her entire set of teeth and successfully rebuilt the bone at the same time. We also put in the implants on the same day. Essentially, we performed three procedures at once.

Sometimes my team and I are even able to do four procedures at once: I will actually put temporary teeth on top of the implants. This means the patient will walk out of the office, the same day that he or she had surgery, with a brand-new smile. By going this route, I preserve as much bone as possible because I do not allow the bone to shrink after removing the teeth. This is a huge psychological lift for patients who are extremely wary of removable dentures. They walk out right after the surgery with their temporary teeth. I typically leave everything in the mouth to heal for a period of four, five, or six months. During that entire time, the patient has a mouth full of natural-looking, temporary teeth. At the end of the healing period, my team and I install the permanent teeth. This process bypasses the many months of healing that have been required traditionally (and as recently as ten years ago).

Certain segments of the population are not good candidates for this procedure, as I discussed earlier. My team and I can still do implants on many of them, but the process may take more time. Allowing for the exception of this minority, I want to explain what each patient can typically expect on the day he or she receives the implants.

What to Expect on Your New-Smile Day

The night before your implant procedure, you will need to avoid eating after midnight because of the IV sedation involved in most procedures. (If I am only doing one or two implants, I usually do not sedate the patient. Most patients do just fine with local anesthesia to prevent pain). That morning, you will take some prescribed medications—usually an anti-inflammatory and a steroid, which will "pretreat" you against postsurgical discomfort, and an antibiotic, which will reduce odds of infection. You will need someone to drive you to the office and back home again afterward. Once you arrive, you will be taken back to the surgical suite where the procedure will actually be performed.

We will make you comfortable in the surgical suite, and then we will connect you to equipment that will monitor your heart rate and respiration. We will also insert the IV lines that deliver sedatives that will be used during your surgery. These sedatives will put you in a state of twilight-conscious sedation. In this state, you will be able to follow simple instructions that allow me to access the areas of the mouth (for example, if I ask you to open your mouth a bit wider, or turn your head toward me, you can do so). Afterward, you will not remember doing this. In fact, you will have complete amnesia regarding the entire procedure. Of course, we will also administer anesthesia, so you will not experience any discomfort during the surgery itself.

After you have been properly sedated and anesthetized, I will remove any teeth that need to be replaced. I will then gently push the gum out of the way to create an *osteotomy*, or a small hole drilled in the jawbone into which the implant itself will be placed, for each implant. I will then put the implants into position, and I will then place small sutures in the gum tissue around the implants' posts. That is it. The implant procedure itself is actually very simple.

Once all your implants have been set properly in place, we will move on to the temporary-teeth stage. As I mentioned before, it is very important to me—and very important to my patients—that no one leaves the surgical suite with visible missing teeth. In some cases, I will place temporary caps on the implant posts. If you are not a candidate for temporary caps, for example, I will modify your existing dentures so you can wear them after the surgery, while your healing is taking place. Typically, I put a cushiony material on the side of your denture that rests against the gums, fitting it so it does not damage the denture or cause you any discomfort. No matter what method I use, you will go home with a smile that same day!

CHAPTER
seven

Your New Life with Your New Smile

Your New Life with Your New Smile

Once I have finished the implant procedure and the patient has been driven home, I typically follow up with him or her the same night of the surgery to make sure the patient is comfortable and doing well. I encourage all my patients to call the office if they need anything. I also give them my cell phone number, along with the assurance that if they feel the need to contact me after hours, they can. Believe it or not, I rarely get calls from patients while they are healing. However, it is important to me that my patients know I am accessible. I want them to feel comfortable, knowing they have my number just in case.

I consider the first week after implant placement to be the most fragile time. This is when the patient's gums start to heal and the bone begins to fuse together. All the bacteria that had been present prior to having the teeth removed are actually being diminished. In terms of recovery, though, the second day is probably the hardest for the patient. After that, recovery becomes easier and easier.

To be honest, patients do have to get over some humps. Some feel practically nothing after their implants. I just saw a patient who had had surgery two days before. She had absolutely no pain afterward. It is great when I have patients like that. I have done extensive work on them and they have experienced no discomfort at all.

Is that standard? To be truthful, no. Most patients can expect some level of discomfort, especially if they have multiple teeth removed. I am honest. I tell patients, "You are going to have some discomfort, but we're going to control it." Through our protocols, we control that discomfort, and we make sure the patient heals properly and goes through the post-surgical stage without problems or complications.

I can prescribe a variety of medications to reduce swelling and alleviate discomfort. I prescribe patients appropriate medication before they leave the office on their "new-smile day." When I check in with them later that evening, I can adjust those medications as needed. I also instruct patients to take vitamin C for a week or two prior to the surgery and for another month afterward. In medical studies, researchers have shown vitamin C assists in the healing process, and good healing is the major goal following any surgery.

I have also found that the ideal eating habits during recovery require a little adjustment on the patients' part. I instruct them to eat a soft diet, typically nothing harder than pasta, for that critical first week. For a single implant, one week is enough. For a full arch implant placement (replacement of all teeth in the upper or lower jaw) I typically recommend that patients continue the softer diet for the entire healing period of three to six months. I warn them that they may lose a few pounds. Most patients giggle and are actually happy with that! Most of my patients do very well on this diet and stick to it beautifully.

I see my patients for follow-up appointments two or three days after they have gotten their implants. This follow-up appointment lets me check to see that they are healing properly. I can also make any necessary adjustments. When patients leave the office the day of their surgery, their mouths still feel numb, so they cannot tell me with 100 percent accuracy how their teeth really feel. This visit gives me an opportunity to check on such things. If a modified denture does not feel just right, or if the bite is a little off, for example, I can fix it. The appointment also serves to reassure the patients that I am still there for them, and if anything looks the least bit abnormal, we will address it.

Two weeks after the surgery, I have each patient come in for another appointment. At that time, I take the gum sutures out, and I check again to make sure that healing is progressing on schedule. By this time in the process, most patients are doing extremely well. For some, the experience is close to miraculous.

For instance, I just saw a patient who had two decayed teeth, one of which had decayed into the root and was causing her pain. The other tooth was loose because her bite had become uneven, thus exerting pressure on that tooth. She was already missing three other teeth and had a partial denture. In a single visit, I removed these two decayed teeth, put in a total of five implants, and cemented temporary teeth over those implants. That patient just came in for her first follow-up. Not only did she have no pain, she was ecstatic that she did not have to wear her partial denture any more. Ten days after the follow-up, I will take her sutures out. Her healing will be complete in about four months.

Three to six months is the typical timeframe for healing after implants. However, I do not wait that long before seeing the patient again. I like to have each patient come in around the two- to three-month mark, about halfway through the healing period, to make sure everything is progressing well and there are no complications. I always tell patients, "If you feel anything that you think is out of the ordinary at any point in the process, do not wait until your next appointment to address it." From the start, I want patients to be clear that they should come right in and let me take a look at any concerns. It is far better to be safe and address problems immediately, as they can often be corrected. I would much rather do that than wait four months to find out about a problem, only to have to tell the patient, "I'm sorry, but your implant has failed. You should have called me sooner."

During the healing period, the bone actually fuses with the implant. The profession has a fancy term for that: *osteointegration*. During the osteointegration, a strong bond forms between the bone and the implant, which makes the implant act as an anchor. When the osteointegration is complete, I will fabricate the teeth over the implant and make the permanent teeth. By this time, the patient's gums will have also healed properly. They will be even and pink in color, with no hint of inflammation or redness.

When I make the permanent teeth, I follow several steps. One thing you should know about me: I take my time in making these teeth. I do not like to rush the process because the permanent teeth— as prosthetics that are going to last ten, fifteen, or even thirty-plus years—are going to be in the patient's mouth for a very long time. As I said before, I admit to being a perfectionist. I want to make sure that these teeth look terrific and that the patient has a ravishing smile.

Yes, I could do things faster, but I would be sacrificing quality. My patients have every right to demand the highest quality for themselves and to expect it from me. If you look at the big picture, taking an additional two or three weeks to get things right is a small price to pay for the end result: a wonderful smile that the patient has had a say in making. Thus, I do not just make the teeth in one visit. I have patients come in two or three times to modify their teeth until we get the smile to the precise stage at which the patient is happy and I am happy. All told, the process of doing this can take anywhere from four to six weeks to finish.

Once we have permanent teeth made to the patient's and my satisfaction, putting them on the implants is very simple. I position them over the implant posts and then cement them in place, just as I would a crown on any tooth. After setting the permanent teeth in the mouth, I make sure that the patient is scheduled for a cleaning appointment in about four weeks' time. My findings at that appointment will serve as an indication of how well the patient is going to care for his or her teeth.

Proper dental care and hygiene is part of my treatment presentation. From the beginning, I tell each patient, "I understand that you have not been to a dentist in thirty years. But if you want to go with this treatment, this is what is going to have to happen: You are going to have to take good care of these new teeth. Otherwise, you are going to compromise everything that we are going to do for you."

My hygienists are very well educated about how to take care of people's teeth, whether those teeth are natural or implants. The hygienists are also extremely skilled at educating patients about how to take care of their teeth at home. I want proper maintenance to begin immediately. That is why, after completing the implant process, we immediately schedule each patient for a complimentary appointment with one of my wonderful hygienists. The purpose of this appointment is to see how good a job the patient is doing and to point out any areas that need improvement. The hygienist will instruct the patient in the proper way of keeping the new teeth clean and give pointers on different tools that can make cleaning easier.

Basically, after you receive your implants, you should treat your new teeth as if they were your natural teeth. You will brush them, floss between them, and use an antibacterial mouthwash just as you would with your natural teeth. With implants, your teeth will not decay, and you will not have cavities. However, as I mentioned previously, you can still suffer from gum problems. Bacteria is what brings most patients to the point at which they need implants, and that bacteria can also cause problems with those implants. This means that just as you must remove the plaque and bacteria from your natural teeth, you must remove the plaque from your implanted teeth. That way, you will not get inflammation in the gums, which can lead to gum disease.

Though we keep it simple, this is vitally important. As I tell my patients, "It is your homework. If you do this part, and we do our part in making sure that we also remove bacteria every time you come here, these teeth should last the rest of your life. But if you disappear, that is when things can go bad."

Luckily, our patients do not disappear. In fact, we see them every three months for the first year following their new smile placement. If they are doing everything right, I extend the time between appointments to every six months in the years after that. I am very proud to say that I have patients for whom I did implants in 1997, and they still come in regularly to have their teeth cleaned and checked. It has been gratifying to see the changes in these people: how they now have healthy, happy smiles in contrast to how they used to live with dentures. It has been equally gratifying for me, as a dentist, to see these people transform from enduring severe states of dental neglect to enjoying their current states. They are proud of their smiles, and they like to take good care of their mouths now. And their self-esteem is amazing.

Years ago, I began a survey of patients on whom I performed implants. Today, nearly one thousand patients have participated in this survey, and I believe its results are a testimony to the wonder of dental implants. Those survey questions and their results are as follows:

- Knowing what you know now, would you have the treatment done again? *98 percent of patients say yes.*

- Was the treatment worth the investment? *98 percent say yes.*

- After treatment, was there a significant improvement in your ability to eat and chew? *97 percent say yes.*

- Was there a significant improvement in appearance? *98 percent say yes.*

- Was there a significant overall improvement? *96 percent said yes.*

As you can see, from the patient's perspective, the success of implants is nothing short of phenomenal. I honestly feel blessed that I have been able to provide them with this success.

Most of my patients make a significant investment in their mouths, so I give them peace of mind that they are making a sound investment with the warranty I offer. After placing more than one thousand implants, I now know that my patients will have no issues whatsoever with their new teeth as long as they come in on a regular basis for cleaning. As a result, I have been able to offer them a five-year warranty on their new teeth and implants. This warranty is contingent on their keeping up with their maintenance and cleaning appointments. If they do not do so, the warranty is voided.

CHAPTER
eight

Money Matters

Implant Costs and Benefits

Money Matters

Implant Costs and Benefits

Dental implants can be a significant investment. Before committing to any investment, you should always consider its costs and benefits carefully. This means taking into account its monetary cost, under what terms those costs can be paid, what you receive in exchange, and what the alternatives are.

Most people find that the increased confidence, enhanced appearance, and vastly improved function provided by secure, implant-supported teeth more than offsets the relatively minor discomfort and inconvenience associated with the implant procedure. Aside from its longevity and decay-proof nature, an implant is largely indistinguishable from a natural perfect tooth. An implant can last the rest of your life. Given the proper care and maintenance, it can be a one-time, lifetime investment.

The initial cost of a dental implant is higher than traditional restoration methods, such as the bridges, partials, and dentures we have already discussed. In general, a patient of mine can expect to pay about $3,000 for a single implant. For a full set of implants, both top and bottom teeth, costs can range from $15,000 to $40,000. These are current cost estimates, and they often change. For example, the price of dental materials has been rising markedly in recent years, and its price can affect total treatment costs.

It is also important to bear in mind that fees for this unique service can vary significantly from individual to individual. Why? Because everyone is different. Just as each person has a different fingerprint, you have a different need than anyone else. Even if you are having a seemingly similar service to that of another patient (for example, suppose you are both having two teeth removed and replaced with implants), your costs will not be identical. Implant dentistry is not a one-size-fits-all service. This makes it impossible to quote a fee for any patient without comprehensive examination and evaluation. Each patient's unique needs, wants, and desires are too variable.

Compared to national averages, the estimates I have given above are competitive. My services are not the most expensive in the country. They are also not the cheapest, and I do not apologize for that. As I have said before, I do not cut corners on my patients' care. Doing so would mean sacrificing quality in terms of the materials, lab services, and highly skilled team I use. Ultimately, this would mean compromising on the quality of the end result I achieve for my patients.

My patients may start out as patients, but as we work together, we become friends. They are truly nice people who have often endured some very unfortunate circumstances that prevented them from being able to take proper care of their mouths. I do not judge them, and I want to make sure they get the best treatment possible. I end up being friends with them because I have their best interests at heart.

The other day I saw one of those friends, a sweet lady who has been a patient of mine for the past ten years and has had implants for almost that long. She had just turned seventy-two, so I sent her flowers to mark the occasion. She came into the office for an appointment shortly after that, and she was so tickled by those flowers. She was very happy, and seeing her that way made my day.

This is the kind of mutual appreciation that marks my relationships with my patients. I appreciate who they are and how they have committed to improving their oral health. In turn, they appreciate who I am and the kind of work that I provide. These relationships are based on respect and trust, and they are fundamental to my practice. I am not looking for a patient who is interested in reducing everything I stand for to the lowest possible dollar amount or the closest possible date. Patients who are simply looking for bargains and/or rush jobs are typically trouble.

As I stated earlier, I realize that implants are a significant monetary investment. My team devotes a great deal of time and effort to ensuring that our patients have a range of financing plans open to them. Since the process of permanent dental implanting takes place in a series of steps over time, your investment can be spread out as long as payment is complete when the work is finished. My office has several third-party financing companies that cater to my patients. These companies offer options that range from twelve- or eighteen-month financing with zero interest to plans that allow for repayment over seven years at low interest rates. In the case of the interest plans, my office does not set the terms. These plans work similar to other types of loans or mortgages: The third-party companies set the interest and terms with the patient, and it is the company that ends up paying my office. The patient then pays the company in accordance with whatever up-front terms have been arranged between the two parties. My team also has different ways to enable financing, such as using 401k plans, insurance, or life insurance value. We can even help patients acquire credit from local banking institutions.

Of course, we accept many forms of dental insurance. However, patients often are not aware that, by and large, dental insurance does not cover implant costs. Despite the fact that dental implants are often a necessity, insurance companies still view them as cosmetic procedures. This means that most dental and medical insurance providers will not cover implants. The insurance situation is getting better, however, in the sense that some dental insurance plans will now cover part of the implant procedure. For example, some insurance providers now allow benefits to be applied to the cost of installing the teeth that go on top of the implants. However, coverage is a decision that rests with one's employer. If the employer is willing to pay for the additional coverage of including part of the implant procedure, the employee will have it. More companies are making this decision. For instance, the Ford Motor Company, in Michigan, just started providing an implant benefit to all its workers. Before 2012, that benefit was not available.

What has not changed, however, is the amount of dental insurance coverage allotted per patient, per year. In 1972, when providers began offering dental insurance, the average policy had a $1,000 limit per year, which means the maximum dollar amount the policy would pay for any and all allowable dental work was $1,000 per year. Today, forty years later, if that amount had merely kept pace with the 3 percent annual inflation rate, the current payment limit would have risen to the neighborhood of $7,000 to $10,000 per year. But guess where the insurance companies are today? They are still offering $1,000 to $1,500.

Here we are, forty years later, with the costs of living going up for patients, and the costs of materials, lab work, employing staff, and hundreds of other aspects of treatment going up for dentists. Yet insurance allowances have largely remained the same. As a consequence, patients will run through their benefits much more quickly than they would have forty years ago. (This is one of the reasons why so many people nationwide have a great deal of incomplete dental work). What's more, insurance premiums continue to increase every year, even as insurance companies keep adding restrictions and limitations to the procedures that patients need and that we dentists need to perform.

Clearly, insurance coverage is a frustrating topic for me. I know it is a frustrating one for my patients as well. However, the bottom line is this: Unfortunately, dental insurance is not like medical insurance, which typically covers a substantial amount of treatment costs. My team will absolutely make every effort to maximize the benefits of our patients' insurance, but it is best for patients to view any dental insurance they have as a form of dental scholarship. It is a nice bonus that takes a bit of the weight off.

Of course, there are things we can do to ease the patients' financial concerns even more, such as staging care. This means we can take care of one section of the mouth—say, put implants in the upper jaw—one year and then do the lower jaw the following year. There are some scenarios, though, in which staging is not possible. If a patient has gum infections in both the upper and lower jaws, and the teeth are considered hopeless, for example, I will shy away from putting the implants in one arch and not the other. I have a very good reason for this: If I put the implants in the upper jaw and the lower jaw still has gum infection, that infection will spread to the upper jaw, thereby creating problems with the implants the patient and I have already invested our time, effort, and money in. Yet again, this is something I will not do because it is not in my patient's best interests.

When it comes to figuring out financing solutions for dental procedures, my motto is, "Where there is a will, there is a way." Finding that way is a matter of figuring out what the best scenario is for the patient, based on each person's financial situation and the care and treatment needed. I understand that costs are a serious consideration for the patient. That is why my team and I work with each patient every step of the way. We address general costs from the first appointment. Based on what we know initially, we can only provide a general range of costs. However, as we actually go through the diagnostic process and learn what each individual's treatment options are, we can provide a more accurate estimate of costs. Then, at the third appointment, we give the patient a firm price based on his or her needs and the final desired outcome. At that time, my team will work with the patient to address the financial concerns involved in the final decision he or she must make. Once the patient reaches a decision about what treatment to pursue, my team and I are ready to help with the financing that will make it happen.

After considering what an implant investment will cost, and the terms under which it can be paid, it is time to look at what the patient will receive in exchange. That involves looking back through this book, which is largely devoted to the rewards that implants deliver—many of which are beyond price. However, it also involves looking at an aspect of implants that many patients do not realize even exists until they have them done: Implants can actually improve a patient's financial picture over the long haul. This is not an overstatement. It is something I have witnessed many times. One patient told me that in the year after he had his implants put in, he increased his sales by a quarter of a million dollars. Another patient of mine spent years stuck in a job that she hated, making just over $20,000 per year. When she came to see me, she told me one of her motivators for getting implants was landing her dream job, which paid a salary of more than $60,000 a year. As soon as she had taken care of her smile, she applied and got the job immediately. Prior to that point, she had not had the courage to pursue her professional dream.

Will such financial gains happen for you? Truly, I cannot say, since I do not know your unique situation. Professional advancement may not even be a concern for you. However, I can say that whatever your personal goals are, you will be better prepared to meet them when you are confident about your smile. Whether you know it or not, by not pursuing treatment for your dental problems, you are experiencing the backlash of something I noted at the beginning of this chapter: The consideration of your alternatives. When dental problems or accidents have taken away one or more of your teeth, your alternatives to implants are either to do nothing or to pursue traditional restoration methods, such as bridges, partials, and dentures. With these alternatives, you are incurring hidden costs, whether you know it or not.

The Horrible Hidden Costs of Not Pursuing Implants

- The cost of teeth that do not look good. Often, people feel so badly about their teeth that they hide their smiles, or stop smiling and laughing altogether.

- The cost of tender gums and constantly uncomfortable or sensitive teeth

- The cost of losing the ability to enjoy your favorite foods

- The cost of worsened nutrition, since you cannot eat a full range of healthy foods

- The cost of outright pain every time you bite down

- The cost of lost self-confidence

- The cost of social withdrawal: avoiding family, friends, and activities you once enjoyed because of social embarrassment

- The cost of romance snuffed out: losing the attention of that certain someone you wanted to notice you

- The cost of losing the job promotion that should have been yours (and the increased earnings that went along with it)

- The cost of ever-increasing unsightly gaps among your teeth that worsen as you age, causing self-esteem to worsen over time in the bargain

- The cost to your whole-body health, including heart attack risks that climb two- to fourfold, worsened diabetes, and/or arthritis that will not get better

- The cost of increasingly depleted physical energy

- The cost of losing your zest for life

- The cost of anxiety over the ever-worsening state of your mouth. For some people, this deepens into depression, a black cloud hanging over your life that will not go away

I don't want you to ever have to pay any of these personal costs, but you may be paying them already. Even if you are not, the longer you wait, the higher the odds are that you will incur one (or many more) of these costs. In my opinion, the costs of not getting dental implant treatment are far higher that the monetary cost of dental implants themselves.

I am not the only person who feels this way. I have heard firsthand from patient after patient about how glad they are they "went for it," and about how they now know what a sound investment they have made. Moreover, I have seen firsthand the life-changing transformations these people have experienced as a result of these implants. I have seen people who were once timid and self-conscious become bubbly and constantly smiling. I have seen people who were constantly passed over at work—and in life—get terrific new jobs and form wonderful new relationships. Over and over, someone who used to be a sad person with low self-esteem ends up being a happier, more functional person. Someone who used to be introverted goes on to become an outgoing individual with more joy in life.

When I started in implant dentistry, I was excited about its promise. I knew that in choosing to make it my specialty, I could make a positive difference in my patients' lives. But I did not realize how amazing that difference would be—nor, to be honest, did I understand what a difference it would make in my life. Seeing patients' newfound confidence, self-esteem, and happiness, as well as receiving their gifts of loyalty and friendship toward me, makes the work I do more rewarding than I ever dreamed.

For you, as a patient, I want more than you ever dreamed. I want you to get the rewards of the Dr. Bazzi Method™, and I want you to experience life as you should. I hope that you will give me the opportunity to provide you with these benefits. Do not let those little voices inside your head cast doubt that stops you. Do not let those little voices make you feel too embarrassed or too afraid to pursue treatment. Take charge and get the new smile you deserve.

For More Information

I invite future patients, their families, and their friends to visit my practice's website at www.contemporarydental.com, and the website I have dedicated specifically to implants, www.dentalimplantsmi.com. Like my practice, the sites are constantly evolving. Still, they always contain up-to-date information about my office, its location, and the services my team offers. Of course, you can call also call the office directly at 734-927-9955. We also offer a toll-free hotline: 888-291-4341 (digit code 522). When you call the hotline, you can listen to an informational message, and then leave your name, phone number, and address if you are interested in having us forward additional information to you.

We welcome communication with prospective patients and maintain communication with the patients we have. This means that you are not only free to call us with any questions, but that we can also connect you with another patient who has been through the implant process. Often, that is an excellent way to get some of your questions answered firsthand.

I limit consultations to a specific number of patients, simply because treating current patients, pursuing my ongoing clinical training, and giving back to my community means my schedule stays full. However, I reserve a limited number of appointments for new patients who want the benefits and results of these advanced implant dentistry methods. My team and I have blocked off a few days of the month specifically for new patients.

For more information on implant dentistry in general, I recommend the following websites:

The International Congress of Oral Implantologists (www.icoi.org)

The International Congress of Oral Implantologists (ICOI) is the world's largest dental implant organization and provider of continuing education in the dental implant area. It is an association for the general public as well as for dental professionals, serving general dentists, oral and maxillofacial surgeons, periodontists, prosthodontists, endodontists, orthodontists, laboratory technicians, auxiliaries, industry representatives, researchers, faculty members, and predoctoral and postdoctoral graduate dental students.

I happen to be a diplomate of the ICOI. This higher credentialing status was added to my name due to my training, success rate, and the extensive research and data gathering I do on all my cases. You can find me using the Find a Member Dentist tool on the ICOI's website.

The American Academy of Implant Dentistry (www.aaid-implant.org)

Founded in 1952, the American Academy of Implant Dentistry (AAID) is the oldest organization devoted to implant dentistry. Its members include general dentists, oral and maxillofacial surgeons, periodontists, prosthodontists, endodontists, orthodontists, laboratory technicians, auxiliaries, industry representatives, researchers, faculty members, and predoctoral and postdoctoral graduate dental students. The AAID's stated mission is "to advance the science and practice of implant dentistry through education, research support and to serve as the credentialing standard for implant dentistry for the benefit of mankind."

The website's Patients and Public section is an excellent resource for those who want to learn more about implants. There you will find brief information on implant benefits, before and after photos, and links to other helpful resources.

The Twenty-Five Advantages of the
Dr. Bazzi Method™

1. An outstanding 95 to 97 percent success rate with implant dentistry. My team and I are able to predictably plan and produce an outcome that is highly favorable for our patients. In addition, we are also able to give patients the peace of mind that the implants they are receiving will last a very long time and will not present them with hassles or future issues.

2. Our dentists are physicians of the mouth. We approach the comfort, health, function, and longevity of each patient's teeth, gums, jaw joint, and chewing mechanism from a solid scientific stance. We base our treatments on dental principles that have been tested over time, and then we improve on them by incorporating the latest breakthroughs in dental research.

3. Treating the patient *as a person*. This is our top priority. Of course, we employ the best treatment practices, which we have learned over years of experience in the field of dentistry. However, just as importantly, we treat each patient with a spirit of warmth and caring, just as we ourselves would like to be treated.

4. Refusal to compromise on treatment. We consider every aspect of how to make each patient's teeth look their best, function properly, and keep their owner healthy. We replace missing teeth with those that are carefully engineered so the recipients look their best and can chew food properly. Enhanced chewing efficiency following implant placement can improve the digestive process. In fact, patients often report a marked reduction in, or resolution of, gastrointestinal problems.

5. The recognition that each patient is unique. We use our experience and know-how to solve each person's dental problems in a way that works for him or her. No patient is ever a textbook case. We carefully customize and carry out each patient's treatment plan according to his or her unique needs. We understand everyone is different. We all have different lives, circumstances, and priorities that play into what constitutes the best care for us. With this understanding, we develop each patient's solutions differently.

6. An advanced, intelligent system of diagnosis and treatment. Through a careful series of consultative, diagnostic, and treatment appointments, we are able to gather all our findings, determine viable courses of treatment, and help patients determine the customized course best for them. We are extremely good at picking out the little treatment details, things one person may require that another person may not.

7. A commitment to never settling for anything but the best for our patients. Our demanding principles translate into great daily challenges, but they are challenges my team and I embrace. We will give each patient a range of treatment options, but we refuse to include any bad options. I have encountered patients who, for one reason or another, have wanted to pursue a treatment that I have not been comfortable doing, not for lack of expertise but because my expertise tells me that the treatment either will eventually fail or will not actually help the patient. I will not pursue a poor course of treatment with anyone. I refuse to recommend anything that will compromise the patient's health.

8. Our full use of the finest cutting-edge techniques and technology. In addition to the top-notch initial education and training I have received, my team and I avidly pursue continuing education. We are always up-to-date with everything that might improve a technique or a service in one way or another. We embrace advancements in the fast-moving field of dentistry. At the same time, however, we make sure that whatever advancements we bring to our office are true improvements that produce predictable, positive results and put each patient's best interests first.

9. A system of care that evolves as the patients' needs do. The implant services we offer are designed to deliver great treatment results: enhanced comfort, reduced anxiety, and a radiant smile. Once those results are achieved, we do not leave the patient behind. Many of our patients

have extensive dental work done, and we want to make sure they are well taken care of afterward. Care does not stop once a patient receives his or her teeth. To ensure each patient great results over the long term, the care we provide evolves to meet each individual's changing needs. We establish a caring, welcoming relationship with each patient that helps ensure he or she will make dental care a personal priority. We want patients to come back to us for regular appointments, and we want them to take care of their teeth at home. We are here to educate patients, answer questions, and address any concerns—now and in the future.

10. Constant attention to maintain and improve the quality of our services. We regularly assess and reassess this quality, and we use these assessments to enhance our patients' experiences. I have spent more than fourteen years conducting an ongoing survey and study of my clinical practice, and I devote untold sums and thousands of hours to additional training and research to go beyond what is required of a dentist. My commitment to improving the quality of my practice, and to increasing my knowledge and skills in the field of dentistry, continues today. It will continue well into the future.

11. The artistic pursuit of beautiful teeth and gorgeous smiles. Again, every patient has different goals in mind. Some want to have beautiful white teeth, while some actually desire less-than-perfect teeth. To me, dental restoration is more than an exacting science. It is a form of art. As

a perfectionist in both my science and my craft, I give attention to every detail. I also take the time necessary to create the ultimate result for each patient.

12. Access to the full range of dental services we offer. In addition to dental implants, we meet a variety of associated oral health needs. We provide typical restorative dentistry to fight gum disease. We offer advanced services that cover the entire scope of general dentistry, including orthodontics, veneer treatment, advanced laser diagnostics, bad breath evaluation, FDA-approved devices for migraine prevention, teeth whitening, and many other services. Through all these services, we provide dental care that significantly impacts people's lives.

13. Preservation of existing teeth. Instead of using a traditional bridge, which requires the two teeth adjacent to a missing tooth to be ground down, we use an implant to replace the affected tooth—without touching the other teeth. This is an extremely conservative solution that optimizes the health of the entire mouth.

14. Rejuvenation in the form and shape of the face. Unlike dentures, implants restore teeth's natural function, including the role they serve in supporting the lips and cheeks. In many cases, a facelift is a happy byproduct of dental implant treatment. In fact, implant restoration can remove ten to fifteen years of age from a patient's appearance. We are putting the teeth back where they are supposed to be. As a consequence, wrinkles are either

eliminated or decreased to the extent that they no longer show.

15. A gorgeous smile! I can't emphasize that enough. When we are placing a full set of implants, we are actually designing a patient's smile from the ground up. We have more say in creating perfection than we do when dealing with someone's natural teeth. The great thing about this is that the implants look entirely real, so only the patient, my staff, and I will know that the patient has teeth that are supported by dental implants.

16. Restored chewing ability. People with dental implants can eat just as they would with a full set of natural teeth. People with dentures or decayed or missing teeth have reduced bite pressure, which limits the foods they are able to enjoy. With implants, their bite pressure returns to normal functioning levels. This means people are able once again to chew a steak, eat corn on the cob, or bite into an apple. They can enjoy all the nutritious foods that they have been missing because of chewing problems brought on by dentures or decayed teeth.

17. Resistance to bone loss and its devastating impact. When someone experiences facial bone loss, his or her natural aging process is going to increase. By putting implants in that person's mouth, we prevent the bone loss that occurs when teeth are lost. In addition, we prevent the accelerated bone loss that can occur when dentures cause gum inflammation. Because implants allow people to

apply natural pressure to underlying bone, and bone is stimulated under that pressure, aging is arrested. People with implants can retain facial bone mass for a longer period of time.

18. Relief from the pain of dentures and partials. Dentures and partials rest on gum tissue, causing inflammation and even chronic sores. People with implants no longer need to suffer from these consequences because the prosthetic teeth are no longer sitting on the gums. Instead, they are sitting on top of the implants, which are imbedded in bone. As long as patients take proper care of their new teeth, implants will not cause long-term damage to gums. Instead, they will improve gum health.

19. An end to embarrassing accidents caused by free-floating dentures. People with implants do not have removable teeth any more. Instead, their teeth are considered *fixed*, which means they are always anchored firmly in the mouth. People with permanent implants go to sleep with their teeth in their mouths and wake up the same way. When speaking to a friend, a colleague, or a family member, or when sitting down to enjoy a meal, people with implants do not have to worry about their teeth falling out.

20. Increased zest for life. By increasing our patients' confidence level, we enable them to begin enjoying themselves again, socializing and experiencing everything that life has to offer.

21. Getting noticed by that special someone. Again, a smile is extremely attractive to the opposite sex. For many patients, just being able to show off their new smiles to people who might not have noticed them in the past is extremely gratifying.

22. Many more smiles. One patient told me, "My cheek muscles are starting to hurt."

    I asked, "Why?"

    She told me, "Well, I am smiling all the time now, and my muscles started to hurt. I am not used to them being worked so hard."

    The two of us chuckled about it, but that made me feel like a million dollars. It was gratifying for me to hear that. If my patients are going to have a problem, that is the kind of problem I can live with them having.

23. Prevention of a bad situation becoming worse. Those who use traditional dentistry methods to replace a lost tooth will get a bridge, which fails after ten years. At that point, they get another bridge, which fails after another five to ten years. Then they get a partial. This creates a domino effect. Today, when people lose a tooth and replace it with an implant, they do not have to worry about damaging the adjacent teeth. Using an implant stops that downward process from getting worse over a period of time. They will not have to go from a bridge to a partial, and then to a denture.

24. A professional payoff. Implants are an investment that pays big dividends every day. In a job setting, people with nice teeth are better perceived and received. People with implants are more likely to get things done the way they want them done, more likely to be rewarded with higher positions, and more likely to receive raises. In business dealings, people with confident smiles have an advantage.

25. A weight of worries lifted from the patient's shoulders and an end to all aspects of dental embarrassment. Many patients are not aware of the options we have for them. It takes a little education to show them what is possible. To this day I am still surprised when a patient tells me, "I didn't know you could do that for me." It can be done, and once it is, people feel it is the best thing they could ever have done.

More Praise from Patients and Fellow Dental Professionals

When I first came into Dr. Bazzi's office, I doubted that anything could be done for me. I had spent years dealing with loose partials and dentures, unable to eat, and hesitant to smile for fear of how my teeth would look. Dr. Bazzi began to tell me what he could do with implants. It all sounded too good to be true, but he did everything he said he would! I cannot even express how I feel now. The comfort is incredible, and I no longer hesitate to smile. I get so many compliments, and it gets better all the time. Thank you, Dr. Bazzi and Contemporary Dentistry.

—Naomi, implant and sedation dentistry patient

Even though I knew it was complex, my treatment seemed simple to me. I was one of those patients who were fearful beyond belief, but Dr. Bazzi's sedation techniques took care of all of that. I went back to work very quickly and without any pain. Things turned out the way I expected, based on how Dr. Bazzi worked with my personal timeframe and without any disruption to my family. I would recommend Dr. Bazzi's implant care to anyone considering it.

—Ellen, implant and sedation dentistry patient

When I had false teeth, there were a lot of foods I couldn't eat, such as corn on the cob. Now I can eat whatever I want thanks to my implants, which are like real teeth. I do not remember a thing from my surgery. It went well with not too much discomfort. It was worth it. Thanks to Dr. Bazzi, my teeth do not fall out in the swimming pool anymore!

—Norm, implant, sedation, and cosmetic denture patient

For the first time in twenty years, I am comfortable enough to be in family photos. Before, I always volunteered to take the photo, since I was so embarrassed about my teeth. Now my teeth look so great everyone thinks they are real. Thanks, Dr. Bazzi!

—Diana, implant and sedation dentistry patient

I would highly recommend Dr. Bazzi for the exceptional skill and patient care he provides. He treats his patients with the utmost dedication, and his results are marvelous. I feel he is the premier dentist to go to in order to restore your smile.

—Dr. Danny Lesser, DDS

I personally recommend Dr. Bazzi as someone to whom to entrust your health and care. Dr. Bazzi cares deeply about each patient and treats each with respect and kindness. He will calm your fears, and he will also provide you with a beautiful smile and a long-lasting solution to your dental concerns.

—Dr. Nathan D. Call, DDS

Dr. Bazzi is one of the most highly skilled dentists I know. He has taken continuing education courses from some of the top professionals in the dental field. Dr. Bazzi and his staff offer dental care in a relaxed, comfortable, and state-of-the-art atmosphere. Dr. Bazzi has a gentle demeanor and a deep understanding of the patient's wants and needs.

He believes in the importance of preventive dentistry and therefore gives very comprehensive dental physicals. All of this helps to make him an exceptional clinician. In his office, smiles are created in the most technical and artistic manner. Many people leave his office "all smiles" with their lives changed.

—Dr. Arnold Kieles, DDS

Canton is fortunate to be home to one of the most skilled dentists in Michigan. Dr. Bazzi has sought training from the most qualified dental professionals in the United States. You will receive the best treatment customized especially for you. He has years of experience rebuilding smiles. You are privileged to have a close-at-hand, talented, caring, gentle dentist who will transform your life by giving you back the confidence and way of life you deserve.

—Dr. Gordon, DDS.

When I first began treatment with Dr. Bazzi I had already undergone major oral surgery and was wearing a full upper denture and a partial lower denture. I originally approached Dr. Bazzi about the process of obtaining dental implants and Dr. Bazzi was very thorough in his explanation of what the procedure entailed. We discussed the benefits of proceeding with the surgery but I was unsure of what to do because of the cost involved and ongoing medical problems I was having. I decided to wait to make sure my medical condition was improved and that I would not have any adverse effects following the procedure. Dr. Bazzi was great in that he did not pressure me but provided me with the necessary information to make an informed decision when I was ready.

One of the things that stuck with me was Dr. Bazzi's statement that obtaining the implants would improve my quality of life and aid in retaining the bone structure of my jaw. I was a little apprehensive about the cost but when I weighed the inconvenience of wearing dentures including not being able to fully taste the food I was eating I decided it was a good idea to begin the process.

We began with the placement of the lower implants which Dr. Bazzi performed in his office without any complications. In fact, I was surprised by how smoothly everything went including minimal swelling and pain afterwards. During my follow-up appointments Dr. Bazzi made sure that the implants were being integrated into the bone and began the process of providing me with new permanent teeth. I really appreciate that he wanted to make sure everything was right and I was happy. Now one year later, I have begun the process all over again with upper implants. I am so excited about the next year and completing this journey with Dr. Bazzi. I am already so much happier since I started this process and would have no problem recommending Dr. Bazzi to family and friends.

If someone had told me that having his dental implant surgery would totally change the quality of my life I would have done it much, much sooner. While it has been a journey for me I recognize that the right time and the right person was available to me and that made the process so much better. Dr. Bazzi's confident, caring manner always made me feel like a valued patient and that was one of the main reasons I chose to entrust him to do this work. This was definitely one of the best decisions I have made in my life and money well spent.

—*Francetta Daniels*

Hi, I am Ron and a patient of Dr. Bazzi. I had implants on the top and bottom put in and I thought I should write about my experience. I had the surgery the first week in December 2011 and I followed his instructions fully. I had all the prescriptions filled and started the pills before surgery just like the instructions said. The surgery went well and the recovery went fast as I think Dr. Bazzi is one of the top dentists in Michigan. I had bone grafts on top along with 8 titanium implants that had to heal, and 6 on the bottom with temporary teeth. I think the hardest part was waiting for the healing process to be complete before the porcelain teeth were installed. But here it is July 2012 and the compliments and the use of the teeth are both great. I really like them and highly recommend Dr. Bazzi for any dental work. Chewing bubble gum and eating granny smith apples are fun now. I like the job I had done and I can't thank Dr. Bazzi enough.

—Ron Balko

M-m-m-m chocolate chip cookies with pecans. I bit into this delectable morsel of sweetness and started chewing. Suddenly my senses alerted me that what I was trying to chew was NOT a piece of pecan but my tooth! Oh my God, thank you for not allowing me to swallow it. What's happening to me now? I was still recovering from a brain aneurysm that happened two years ago in 2004. Now I am loosing my teeth. I have to go find a dentist, PRONTO! I was already wearing a flipper, because I had dislodged my front tooth in the late 1980's. I have got to find a dentist PRONTO!

As I normally do on Sundays after church service and dinner, I relax by reading the newspaper. I don't recall what section I was reading at time, but Dr Bazzi's advertisement caught my attention.

Oh goody a dentist that's not far from home, how convenient. I called Monday and made an appointment.

After my initial consultation, Dr Bazzi informed me that I had a couple of issues that needed to be addressed regarding my dental health first before we began the cosmetic work. I was sure I had issues with my dental health, because a couple of years ago I had a craniotomy because of a brain aneurysm and my dental health was not a priority. Dr Bazzi said we here at Contemporary Dentistry will take of you and your dental health issues. But first we must get your gums healthy to do a bone graft to prepare for implants. Bone graft! Yes Dr Bazzi gently said and explained in laymen terms why I needed the bone graft to support the implants. I said okay, because I was so vain I didn't want to place my teeth in a container on the bathroom counter. Great if I am going to go through all of these procedures, I want to have a "Hollywood" smile.

I didn't return until a year later. Why? I was afraid. Because of the aneurysm I did not want to undergo anesthesia again. This would be necessary to do a bone graft. I told Dr Bazzi why I was afraid of being anesthesized, which is why it was taking so long to make a decision about having the procedure to restore my smile. Dr Bazzi than explained the before (prep), during, and after effects of what I would experience. He assured me he had performed this procedure many times, with great results, and he and his competent staff would take care of me.

They did an excellent job, a five star rating job. The next day I received a follow-up care telephone call to be sure I was not having any complications and flowers.

In 2008 I finally received my "hollywood" smile and I am still getting compliments. I am to date a very satisfied patient and friend of Dr Bazzi and his wonderful staff.

Thank you Dr Bazzi and staff for my "HOLLYWOOD" smile.

—Ulace Butler

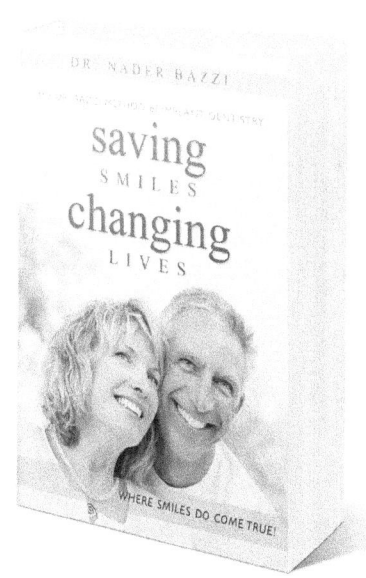

How can you use this book?

MOTIVATE

EDUCATE

THANK

INSPIRE

PROMOTE

CONNECT

Why have a custom version of *Saving Smiles, Changing Lives*?

- Build personal bonds with customers, prospects, employees, donors, and key constituencies
- Develop a long-lasting reminder of your event, milestone, or celebration
- Provide a keepsake that inspires change in behavior and change in lives
- Deliver the ultimate "thank you" gift that remains on coffee tables and bookshelves
- Generate the "wow" factor

Books are thoughtful gifts that provide a genuine sentiment that other promotional items cannot express. They promote employee discussions and interaction, reinforce an event's meaning or location, and they make a lasting impression. Use your book to say "Thank You" and show people that you care.

Saving Smiles, Changing Lives is available in bulk quantities and in customized versions at special discounts for corporate, institutional, and educational purposes. To learn more please contact our Special Sales team at:

1.866.775.1696 • sales@advantageww.com • www.AdvantageSpecialSales.com